Current Topics in Pathology

Continuation of Ergebnisse der Pathologie

72

Editors

C. L. Berry E. Grundmann W. H. Kirsten

Pathology of a Black African Population

By

C. Isaacson

With 82 Figures

Springer-Verlag Berlin Heidelberg New York 1982

C. Isaacson, Professor, The Laboratory, Baragwanath Hospital,
Department of Anatomical Pathology, South African Institute for Medical Research and University of the Witwatersrand, P.O. Box 1038,
Hospital Stredt, Johannesburg 2000, RSA

C.L. Berry, Professor Dr., Department of Morbid Anatomy, The London Hospital Medical College, University of London, London E1 1BB, Great Britain

E. Grundmann, Professor Dr., Pathologisches Institut der Universität, Domagkstraße 17, D-4400 Münster/Westf., Germany

W.H. Kirsten, Professor Dr., Department of Pathology, The University of Chicago, 950 East 59th Street, Chicago, IL 60637, USA

ISBN-13:978-3-642-81800-4 e-ISBN-13:978-3-642-81798-4
DOI: 10.1007/978-3-642-81798-4

Library of Congress Cataloging in Publication Data
Isaacson, C. (Charles), 1929– Pathology of a Black African population. (Current topics in pathology; v. 72) Bibliography: p. Includes index. 1. Blacks–Diseases–South Africa. 2. Urban health–South Africa. 3. Blacks–Diseases–South Africa–Soweto. 4. Urban health–South Africa–Soweto. I. Title. II. Series. RBl. E6 vol. 72 [RA552.S6] 616.07s 82–773 ISBN-13:978-3-642-81800-4 [614.4′268] AACR2

2122/3130–543210

Preface

Various nouns have been used in the past to describe the Black races of South Africa and these terms will be used interchangeably in the text. They include "Bantu, African, Negro and Black". Although the currently recommended term is that of "Blacks of South Africa", many articles have been published in the Medical literature referring to Bantu, e.g., "Bantu Siderosis", and other articles have appeared referring to African, e.g., "African Cardiomyopathy".

The material for this study was derived from the pathology laboratory at Baragwanath Hospital (2,500 beds) which serves the town of Soweto, a Black town of approximately 1 million inhabitants ten miles southwest of Johannesburg. There may, of course be differing incidence rates for various diseases in different parts of South Africa, although the overall trend is fairly uniform. No figures are available as to how long the inhabitants of Soweto have lived in the town or whether a significant percentage originated in rural areas. No comparisons were therefore attempted between disease in rural and urban areas. The material in this book deals essentially with pathology in the urban Black. This book is not a comprehensive study of pathology in the black Community. Only certain aspects are dealt with, particularly those topics of interest to the author. With the process of urbanization and westernization, rapid changes are taking place in the pattern of disease in this population, and it was felt imperative that a book of this nature should document certain disease patterns before they become modified. This is a population in whom hypertension is rampant, although coronary artery occlusion is rare, where a veritable epidemic of oesophageal carcinoma is raging; a population in which, if carcinoma of the cervix could be eliminated, the adult female would not have a major cancer problem, and in which, if carcinoma of the oesophagus and liver could be eliminated, the adult male would not have a significant cancer problem. It is in the Blacks of South Africa in which the fascinating topic of oral iron overload has been most extensively studied. The pattern has changed as a result of the alteration in drinking habits and the free availability of the White man's liquor, and recently alcoholic liver disease akin to that seen in Western societies has become manifest. Many important diseases in the African population such as tuberculosis, amoebiasis, and bilharziasis are not considered.

There are many people who rendered invaluable assistance in this project; my Registrars and the Clinicians associated with much of the material. Particular thanks is due to Mr. D. Treunich, senior technologist in the histopathology laboratory at Baragwanath Hospital, and my secretaries, Miss N.M. Mazamisa and Mrs. L.M. Moloi, who patiently bore the brunt of my impatience. May I express my gratitude to the late Max Ulrich who was responsible for all the photography. Max was taken away from us suddenly at the peak of his career. Apart from his outstanding professional ability, Max was one of God's "gentleman". We miss you Maxie.

This entire work would not have been possible without the moral and financial support of the South African Institute for Medical Research and particularly its able Director, Professor Jack Metz.

Johannesburg *Charles Isaacson*

Contents

Indexed in ISR

Chapter 1

Cardiomyopathy

Introduction

Many papers have appeared from the African continent dealing with types of non-coronary heart failure of unknown aetiology which are rare in the more sophisticated society of the West. The first of these from South Africa was that by *Gillanders* (1951) entitled "Nutritional heart disease," as he felt that malnutrition was of primary aetiological importance. His cases displayed the common signs of congestive failure with enlargement of the whole heart, gallop rhythm and severe oedema and he maintained that liver disease and malnutrition were prime aetiological factors. Subsequently *Higginson* et al. (1952) described the necropsy findings in 12 cases. *Becker* et al. (1953) then described a group of hearts in White and Black subjects which they called "Cardiovascular collagenosis with parietal endocardial thrombosis," and in which they felt that the pathogenesis was basically a disturbance of the connective tissues of the heart, and that, accordingly, the condition should be included in the group of diffuse collagen diseases, along with other well recognized types such as periarteritis nodosa, lupus erythematosus, diffuse scleroderma and rheumatic heart disease.

There seems no doubt that the conditions described independently by *Becker* et al. and *Higginson* et al. are the same entity, and that in South Africa there is one form of idiopathic cardiomyopathy, characterized by hypertrophied, dilated hearts, often with intraluminal thrombi in various stages of organization. Dispute however, exists in relation to pathogenesis. Whereas, *Becker* et al. claimed that the initial insult is directed against the endocardium, *Higginson* et al. felt that the basic lesion is in the myocardium.

Powell and *Wright* (1965) reporting from Durban found that cardiomyopathy constituted 34% of 270 consecutive African male patients in congestive cardiac failure. They maintained that there is a similarity between idiopathic cardiomyopathy and alcoholic heart disease, although they were not able to detect any evidence of alcoholism or malnutrition. *Kallichurum* (1976), contrary to most other investigators, found right ventricular predominance to be common in cardiomyopathy and suggested that pulmonary vasoconstriction, episodic in type, rather than sustained, could be responsible for this and that the cardiac lesions could be explained on the basis of anoxia resulting from coronary vasoconstriction.

Pathology of Idiopathic Cardiomyopathy

Materials and Methods

The most comprehensive description of the pathology of idiopathic cardiomyopathy was that by *Higginson* et al. (1960) and their findings are quoted in detail. They described the necropsy findings in 80 cases derived from 537 cases of heart failure in a total of 2367 necropsies.

In their series idiopathic cardiomyopathy was the fourth commonest cause of death amongst cases of heart failure. At the time it was however, considered the commonest heart disease admitted to the wards. Although the autopsy incidence appears to have dropped, the disease is still frequent (Tables 1.1, 1.2).

Pathological Features

Cardiovascular System

Pericardial sac: A small excess of pale straw-colored fluid is common. Microscopic examination in most cases shows a slight, predominantly lymphocytic infiltration of the epicardium. Rarely, death may result from a haemopericardium due to injury to a markedly thinned right ventricular wall following a clinical diagnosis of pericardial effusion and paracentesis. A clinical diagnosis of pericardial effusion is not infrequent.

Heart

Macroscopic examination: In all cases the heart is hypertrophied and dilated. The hypertrophy is usually generalized and involves all chambers equally. In some cases the enlargement is more marked on the right side whereas in others it is more marked on the left side (Fig. 1.1). The ratio of heart/body weight ranges from 0.5 to 1.0%. The heart weights vary from 300 gm to 800 gm. In more than half the cases intralum-

Table 1.1. Distribution of cardiac diseases at autopsy and their percentage of the total cardiac deaths (*Isaacson* 1977)

	1959	1960	1976
Total	111	122	120
Idiopathic cardiomyopathy	37 (33%)	22 (18%)	17 (14.1%)
Myocardial infarction	1 (0.9%)	1 (0.81%)	14 (11.7%)
Hypertension	43 (40%)	51 (43%)	51 (43.3%)
Syphilitic aortitis	3 (2.7%)	2 (1.6%)	–
Rheumatic heart disease	24 (22%)	33 (27%)	25 (20.8%)
Cor pulmonale	2 (1.8%)	4 (3.2%)	–
Miscellaneous	(1.2%)	(6.4%)	(10%)

Table 1.2. Age and sex distribution of various cardiovascular and renal diseases (*Isaacson* 1977)

Age in years	Total	1–19	20–29	30–39	40–49	50–59	60+	Unknown
Idiopathic cardiomyopathy								
Males	48	4	4	12	11	3	13	1
Females	28	1	3	7	5	7	5	–
Total	76	5	7	19	16	10	18	1
Myocardial infarction								
Males	10	–	–	–	1	5	4	–
Females	6	–	–	–	1	–	5	–
Total	16	–	–	–	2	5	9	–
Essential hypertension								
Males	47	–	2	3	14	12	16	–
Females	66	–	5	11	16	16	18	–
Total	113	–	7	14	30	28	34	–
Hypertension due to chronic glomerulonephritis								
Males	11	2	3	–	3	1	2	–
Females	9	–	1	5	2	1	–	–
Total	20	2	4	5	5	2	2	–
Rheumatic heart disease								
Males	35	6	9	7	6	7	–	–
Females	45	9	5	13	9	5	3	1
Total	80	15	14	20	15	12	3	1

inal thrombi are present. These vary from recent mural thrombi superimposed on an apparently intact endocardium and myocardium to dense organized thrombi forming fibrous plaques obliterating the spaces between the trabeculae carneae. In some cases fibrous bands extend deep to the thrombi into the underlying myocardium, but in the majority the thrombi and the muscle are clearly demarcated (Fig. 1.2). Thrombi are most frequently found in the right atrial appendage and at the apex of the left ventricle, where the underlying myocardium is sometimes partially or completely replaced by fibrous tissue merging with the thrombi. In a few cases slight focal fibrous scarring of the myocardium is observed, apart from fibrosis and degeneration associated with thrombosis.

In occasional hearts thick fibrous plaques are present overlying the endocardium. From the microscopic examination (vide infra) it appears that these represent old organized thrombi. Only rarely does one see endocardial fibrous plaques comparable in extent to that described in Uganda (*Davies* 1948).

No significant valvular lesions are seen in any case. In some hearts the coronary arteries show mild atherosclerosis but in no case is significant diminution of the lumen present, and the degree of atherosclerosis is no greater than that seen in hearts of patients dying from noncardiac disease.

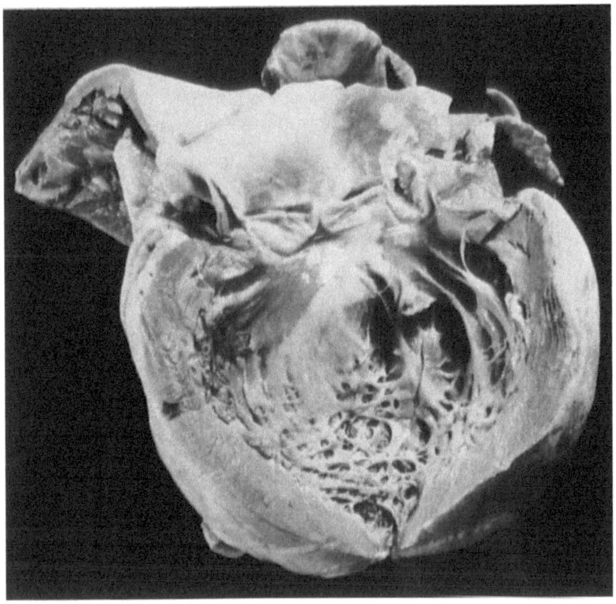

Fig. 1.1. Case of idiopathic heart failure with markedly hypertrophied left ventricle and thickened endocardium

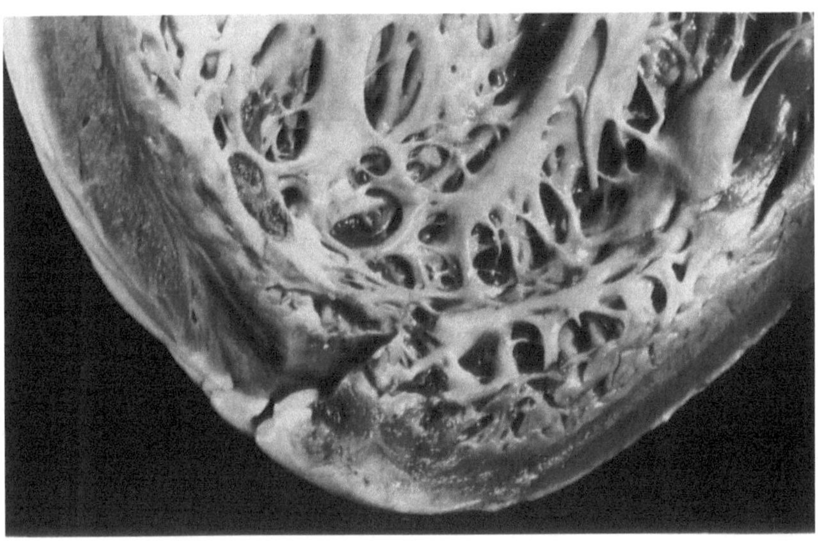

Fig. 1.2. Note the apical thrombi and the marked fibrous endocardial thickening. The fibrous bands extend deeply into the underlying myocardium which is markedly thinned at the apex

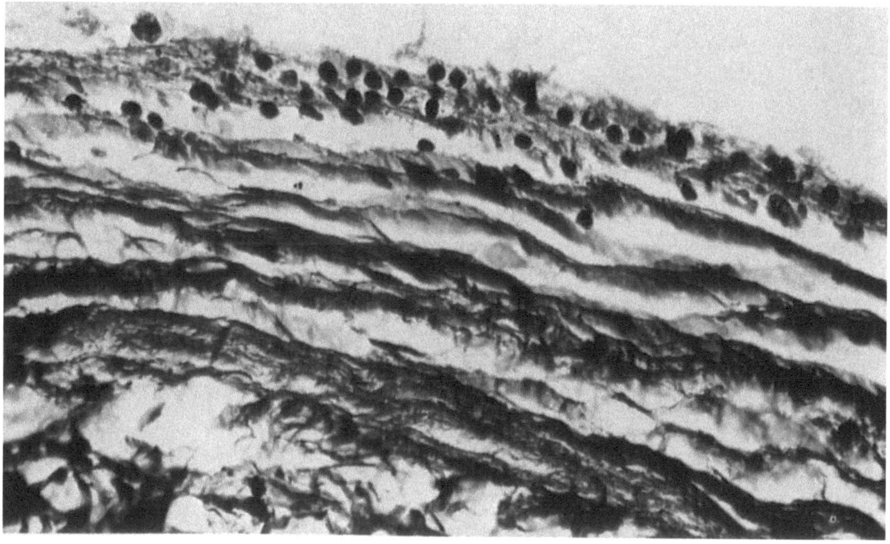

Fig. 1.3. Section of the endocardium showing a focus of infiltration by lymphocytes. H&E, ×370

Microscopic Examination

Endocardial Lesions

The endocardium in the majority of hearts appears normal, but areas of mild nonspecific diffuse and focal thickening are sometimes observed. In about a quarter of the cases small foci of lymphocytes, macrophages, and plasma cells are present in the endocardium (Fig. 1.3).

Significant lesions are present in relation to thrombus formation. In some hearts large bulky recent thrombi can be seen deposited on an apparently normal endocardium (Fig. 1.4). In other areas the thrombi are composed of very small fibrin clots. The thrombi are most frequent between the interstices of the trabeculae carneae and in some cases are also observed arising from or extending into the Thebesian veins. They show all stages of development, some being clearly of recent origin and composed of fibrin clot, whereas others have undergone organization and fibrosis. The deeper portion is usually more fibrosed.

The probable sequence of events is as follows. In the early stages numerous fibroblasts can be seen extending from the endocardium and from the luminal side of the thrombus into the clot, transforming it into a mass of granulation tissue with newly formed capillaries sometimes surrounded by hemosiderin deposits and mildly infiltrated by chronic inflammatory cells. Later the thrombi become transformed into relatively avascular fibrous plaques. Some plaques merge with more recent thrombi on the surface, whereas others are covered by a layer of endothelial cells. The changes can be observed in many parts of the heart but organization tends to be most advanced at the

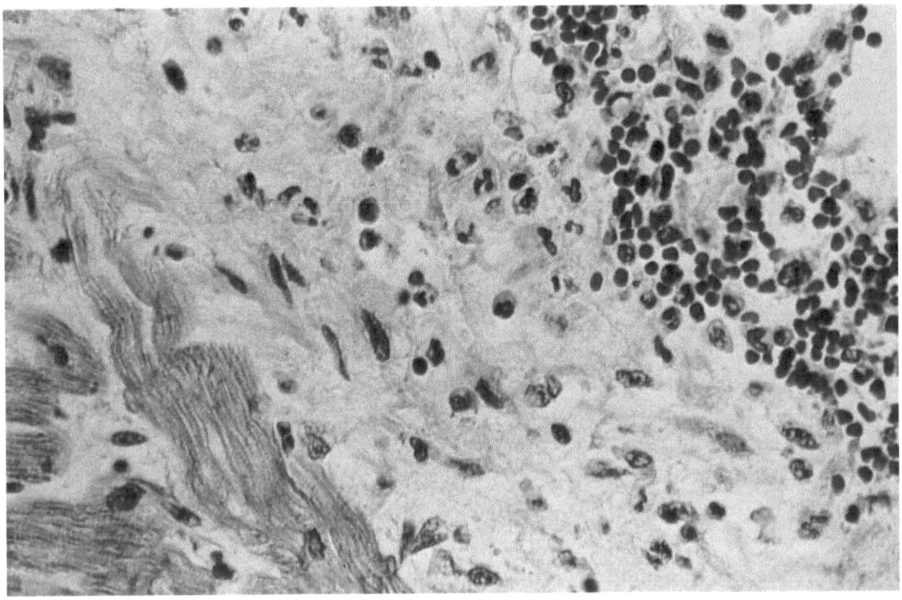

Fig. 1.4. Lymphocytes and neutrophils infiltrating the endocardium at site of attachment to thrombus. H&E, ×370

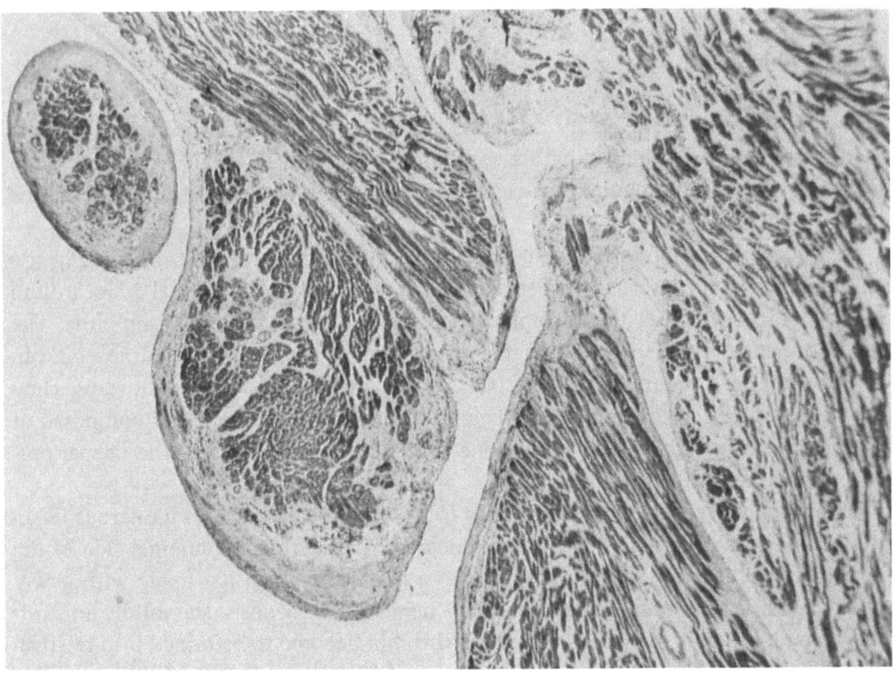

Fig. 1.5. Fibrous thickening of the endocardium of the papillary muscles. H&E, ×26

apex of the left ventricle. In the late stages with well-marked fibrous plaque formation, a few poorly stained elastic fibres are sometimes present, but marked elastic tissue formation is not a feature (Fig. 1.5). Calcification is not seen in contrast to the findings in Uganda.

Myocardium

The myocardium consistently shows hypertrophy of the muscle fibres which contain large "stag-horn" nuclei. Sometimes the fibres show a mild nonspecific intracellular oedema with separation of myofibrils. No parasites or significant hemosiderin deposits are present. In many hearts there is some degree of interstitial oedema between the muscle fibres associated sometimes with deposition of a poorly staining collagenous tissue. Small foci of fibrous scarring are sometimes observed with degeneration of muscle fibres. Such scarring is usually mild but may be more prominent in some cases (Fig. 1.6). Occasionally such foci are associated with scanty lymphocytic infiltration which is always mild. Usually these myocardial lesions are related to the presence of mural thrombi, but in a small percentage of cases scarring can be seen in regions where no thrombi are present and this usually involves the inner third of the myocardium. It is possible that such foci are ischaemic in origin and the result of emboli to the coronary arteries. Surviving muscle fibres can be observed between the scar and the endocardial surface. In papillary muscles and trabeculae carneae covered by organized thrombi, the muscle fibres are often degenerate, showing a "moth-eaten" appearance.

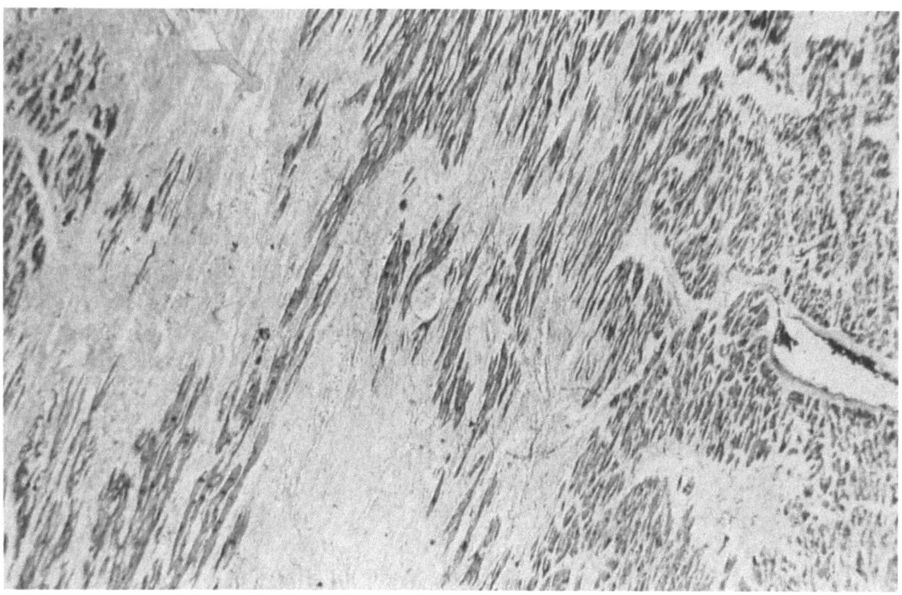

Fig. 1.6. Marked interstitial fibrosis of the myocardium. H&E, ×23

Occasionally similar changes are noted in the absence of thrombi. Fibrosis and myocardial degeneration are also frequently noted in the atria, and may be more marked than in the ventricles.

Vessels

The coronary arteries show varying degrees of atherosclerosis but of no greater severity than in other subjects of similar age. The small myocardial arteries and arterioles show no evidence of fibrinoid necrosis or arteritis.

Other Organs

The serous cavities contain varying quantities of transudate. In all cases there is generalized venous congestion of the lungs, kidneys, spleen and brain. In addition in about one third of the cases there is obvious visceral infarction involving the lungs, kidneys spleen and brain. No evidence of primary lung disease or bilharzial fibrosis of the lungs is found. The kidneys show the normal changes associated with increasing age.

Pathogenesis

Higginsson et al. (1960) suggested that the essential clinical and pathological features indicate that the basic lesion is myocardial weakness, leading to dilatation and hypertrophy, with secondary changes induced by development of mural thrombi. There does not appear to be any correlation between the length of history and the degree of myocardial hypertrophy, and no satisfactory explanation of the aetiology of the myocardial dysfunction and hypertrophy emerges. They also postulated some derangement in the blood dynamics within the heart due to incomplete emptying in systole, and resultant stasis. The fact that the thrombi occur in the atrial appendages or between the trabeculae carneae supports the view that stasis is a factor in their formation. The presence of a pre-existing endocardial lesion is difficult to prove in cases where organization of a thrombus has obscured the relationship of thrombus to endocardium.

Discussion of Aetiology

Nutrition

Gillanders (1951) originally entitled these hearts "Nutritional heart disease" as he felt that malnutrition was of primary aetiological importance. His cases displayed the common signs of congestive failure with enlargement of the whole heart, gallop rhythm and severe oedema, and he also maintained that liver disease was an invariable accompaniment and found that in most cases signs of failure retrogressed when a well balanced diet was substituted for the deficient diet to which patients had being acustomed, and that the disease relapsed when patients left hospital and reverted to their previous diets. He suggested that the ultimate failure of the heart might be conditioned by primary failure of the liver as a result of malnutrition. In support of this theory, *Reid* (1970) was able to produce changes similar to those observed in cardiomyopathy in rats by feeding them on a diet deficient in tryptophan.

Brand et al. (1965) found red cell thiamine concentration was normal in 70% of cardiomyopathy patients, so that in this group thiamine deficiency was not believed to be an aetiological factor. In 18% of the cardiomyopathy patients however, the thiamine concentration was as low as in patients with florid beri-beri, and it was suggested that these were possible examples of atypical beri-beri heart disease. *Falase* et al. (1973) claimed that the Nigerian idiopathic cardiomegaly, also known as heart muscle disease, may in reality be a form of beri-beri heart disease. This was based on assessments of the thiamine nutritional status.

Seftel et al. (1972) accentuated that thiamine deficiency may coexist with other forms of heart disease.

For example, they noted that myocardial failure not infrequently occurs in Blacks with moderate degrees of hypertension, of chronic chest disease etc., and although this had usually been attributed to the coexistence of idiopathic cardiomyopathy, their observations suggested that coexistent thiamine deficiency may also be responsible. In the group of thiamine deficient patients with persistent cardiomegaly, the other important factor inherent in the alcoholic beri-beri situation, namely ethanol excess, may be of significance.

Seftel (1973) clearly distinguished beri-beri heart disease and idiopathic cardiomyopathy. Beri-beri is largely a disease of male migrant manual labourers who live a hostel-type existence and drink heavily. This disorder usually takes the form of reversible high output heart failure, but other syndromes of thiamine deficiency also occur.

Significant myocardial abnormalities have been demonstrated in children with kwashiorkor, including vacuolation, atrophy of myocardial fibres and variation in size of the fibres (*Wharton* et al. 1969). Occasionally apical left ventricular thrombosis has been noted. These may be responsible for functional changes such as a reduction in cardiac output and also a liability to cardiac failure or sudden death during the early phases of treatment. In some fatal cases there are histologic changes resembling those in idiopathic cardiomyopathy. The possibility that idiopathic cardiomyopathy in later life may be a sequel to kwashiorkor has still to be explored.

Alcohol

According to *Brigden* and *Robinson* (1964) there is a close similarity between cardiomyopathy in blacks and the findings in alcoholic heart disease. *Grusin* (1957) in describing the so called acute reversible heart failure in Africans, made it clear that alcoholism is a significant feature in many patients with heart disease admitted to hospital in Johannesburg, and that the response to thiamine may be very variable and may well depend on the chronicity of the heart disease. *Shaper* (1968) came to the conclusion that chronic malnutrition per se is not a significant factor in idiopathic cardiomyopathy in South Africa and that alcohol may play a direct and important role in this disease, particularly in the adult males of all races. There is today a great deal of evidence to show that excessive chronic consumption of ethanol may damage cardiac muscle and produce a cardiomyopathy. The ethanol itself is noxious but it is also likely that the associated malnutrition is contributory. Alcoholism appears to be of central significance in the genesis of a whole spectrum of cardiac conditions in the Johannesburg Blacks. It is undoubtedly the main factor conditioning the development of thiamine deficiency and reversible beri-beri heart disease. In addition, alcohol excess may be cardiopathic in its own right, which may explain the variable behaviour of the myocardium in alcoholic beri-beri, and its association with persistent cardiomegaly. On the basis of clinical, epidemiological and laboratory evidence, *Seftel* et al. (1972) advanced the hypothesis that ethanol excess and/or chronic general malnutrition may explain the majority of cases of idiopathic cardiomyopathy in both males and females. There is more direct evidence to support the aetiology of ethanol in this condition in that the male: female ratio is 3, 3:1 which is in keeping with the sex ratio of drinkers in the city.

In addition, about 30% of male idiopathic cardiomyopathy sufferers show other evidence of ethanol excess including pellagra, acute and chronic scurvy, peripheral neuropathy, severe siderosis and cirrhosis (*Seftel* 1972).

Recent studies by *McPhail* et al. (1979) using the level of iron in the liver and spleen as an indicator of beer consumption, confirm that approximately 50% of all males with idiopathic cardiomyopathy contain significantly more iron in their livers and spleens than the general population, suggesting that in adult males half the cases of idiopathic cardiomyopathy are heavy beer drinkers. Of the females however, very few demonstrated a significantly higher level of iron in the liver and spleen as compared with the general population.

It is however, clear that ethanol excess cannot explain the majority of cases of idiopathic cardiomyopathy, and in half the males and a large proportion of females and in all children, some other factor must be operating, probably malnutrition. Idiopathic cardiomyopathy is common among rural Blacks whose living conditions are poor. Similarly post partum cardiomyopathy, probably a variant of idiopathic cardiomyopathy, results from the interaction of the stresses of the post partum period and and underlying cardiomyopathy and the precipitating stresses and the underlying cardiomyopathy are probably nutritional in origin.

Miscellaneous

In infants and children idiopathic cardiomyopathy is not associated with malnutrition and in this group particularly, a previous myocarditis may be an important factor. *Parry* and *Abrahams* (1965) felt that, because many patients with endomyocardial fibrosis start the disease with an acute initial illness with systemic symptoms, the initial event commonly beginning during the rainy season, the aetiological agent may well be an organism of a vector of disease which is prevalent in the rainy season.

Brockington et al. (1967) reporting a case of endomyocardial fibrosis in a European resident for 15 years in Eastern Nigeria, suggested that the disease is not caused by a genetic characteristic or by malnutrition, but that the distribution and pattern of the disease favour an infective agent. *Bada* (1973) reported 70 cases of idiopathic cardiomyopathy from Liberia and felt that the aetiology was multiple, but suggested the possibility of a low potassium due to malnutrition. *Connor* et al. (1968) in describing endocardial fibrosis in Uganda, suggested that the histological changes observed were consistent with a hypersensitivity mechanism.

None of the cases gave a familial history and there does not appear to be any relationship to the familial cardiomyopathies (*Emmanuel* 1972).

Comparison with Idiopathic Heart Failure in Uganda and Nigeria

In Uganda, endomyocardial fibrosis is a major problem, accounting for about 15% of all cases of heart failure at autopsy (*Davies* 1961). Clinically, these cases may present as bicameral heart failure with either mitral or tricuspid incompetence, more rarely stenosis, or with both atrioventricular valves affected. Some cases mimic constrictive pericarditis, whereas others present with large pleural effusions. Embolic complications are infrequent. In severe cases the heart lesions are striking. There is a massive scarring process involving the apices of the ventricles and the inflow tracts extending to behind the posterior artrioventricular valve leaflets. The result is often fusion of the papillary muscles and chordae tendineae, with sealing of the posterior cusp of the atrioventricular valves to the mural endocardium. The right ventricle may be similarly affected. The whole apex of the right ventricle may become filled with a mass of clot and fibrous tissue.

The scar tissue consists of a superficial layer of hyaline tissue with looser textured fibrous tissue in the deeper layers. These findings are observed in the severe cases but there are all grades of involvement. Many of the subjects show only mild fibrous thickening of the endocardium and histologically these cases are indistinguishable from those seen in South Africa. Some of the differences enumerated by *Davies* (1961) are not all that well defined and many of the clinical and pathological features merge. The severe type of endocardial fibrosis is never seen in South Africa, but apical fibrosis following organization of thrombi is frequent, and histologically such an area may resemble a less severely affected area in a Ugandan-type heart. That there are differences between the two conditions there is no doubt. The South African hearts are usually much larger, generally with ventricular hypertrophy, and apical recession is unknown. The less severely affected Ugandan hearts (and they form a significant percentage) are not very different from those seen in South Africa.

The picture in Nigeria is a little different. *Edington* and *Jackson* (1963) described two main types of idiopathic heart failure; heart muscle disease, and endomyocardial fibrosis. Heart-muscle disease, probably the commonest cardiological lesion in Nigeria, presents a clinical and pathological picture identical with that of the South African cases. They show a characteristic hypokinetic circulation, often with mild hypertension during bouts of failure, oedema, thready pulse and cardiomegaly. Pathologically, too, they resemble the South African cases with large hearts, showing hypertrophy and dilatation affecting all chambers, foci of endocardial thickening and intraluminal thrombi undergoing organization. Like the South African cases, they are not infrequently incorrectly diagnosed as aortic incompetence or pericardial effusion because of the quiet heart sounds and the gross cardiomegaly. The hearts with endomyocardial fibrosis are identical to those seen in Uganda with characteristic distortion and partial obliteration of the ventricles, the white fibrous tissue over the endocardium enmeshing the papillary muscles and encroaching on the posterior cusps of the atrioventricular valves.

The histological appearances of the South African, Ugandan and Nigerian subjects show many features in common. *Edington* and *Jackson* (1963) voice the opinion that the South African idiopathic cardiomyopathy and the Nigerian heart-muscle disease are identical, that these two are closely related to the endomyocardial fibrosis of both Nigeria and Uganda, and that the absence of severe endomyocardial fibrosis in South Africa or in Nigerian heart-muscle disease may be explained by postulating that the latter two myopathies are of a more acute type so that endomyocardial fibrosis is rare. When the condition is more chronic, patients rarely die before the endocardium is severely affected.

Idiopathic Cardiac Hypertrophy in Black Children

In 1956 *Altman* and *Stein* reported four cases of idiopathic cardiac hypertrophy in African children characterized by congestive cardiac failure, with general enlargement of the heart, without a distinct congenital anomaly, or known cardiovascular disease as a cause. Clinically, there was no evidence of rheumatic fever, chronic pulmonary disease, nephritis or anaemia while post mortem examination excluded congenital heart disease, myocarditis, glycogen storage disease, endocardial fibroelastosis and rhabdomyoma. Clinically, the cases closely parallelled *Gillanders'* description of so-called nutritional heart disease or idiopathic cardiomyopathy with the hypokinetic circulation, the poor movement of the heart as seen fluoroscopically, and the poor response to treatment. However, there was no evidence that malnutrition was a casual factor, and in fact, the state of nutrition was much above average in these cases with no evidence of dermatosis, liver disturbance, oedema or other stigmata of malnutrition. Subsequently, *Stein* et al. (1964) reported the detailed pathology of these cases.

There were thirteen boys and ten girls, and the ages ranged from six months to seven years. Only three were under one year of age and there was no family history of a similar affection in any. In none of the children was there any real evidence to suggest that malnutrition was an aetiological factor and thiamine was also administered to several without response. The children all suffered from clinical low output cardiac failure. Most cases had an atrial gallop rhythm and there was a striking absence of significant cardiac murmurs. Radiographs and fluoroscopy showed cardiomegaly and a

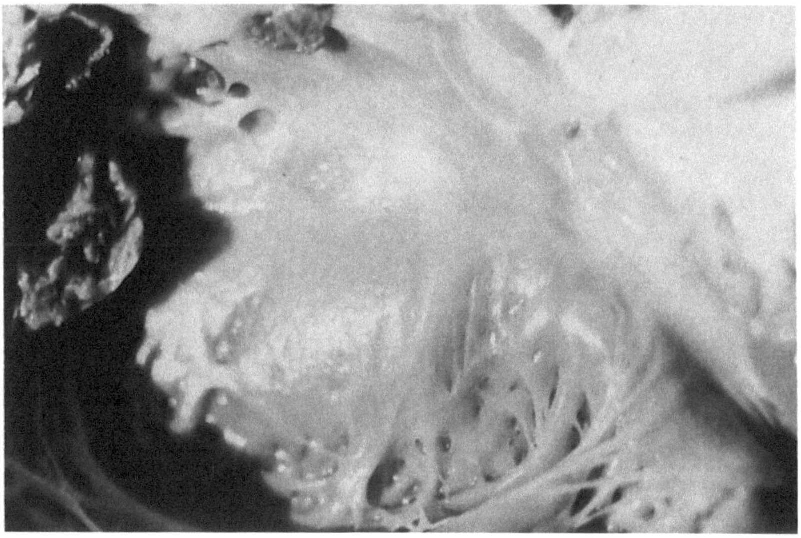

Fig. 1.7. Fibrous thickening of the endocardium of the left ventricle with superimposed mural thrombosis

globular shape to the heart which pulsated very poorly and often suggested a pericardial effusion. However, when the pericardium was tapped no fluid was obtainable. Hemiplegia in four children was due to embolic phenomena. Viral studies, including those for Coxackie virus were all negative. Skeletal muscle biopsy on six patients showed no excess of glycogen.

Pathology

The heart weights range from one and a half to three and a half times the normal. Macroscopically, there is usually hypertrophy and dilatation of both ventricles, the left predominating. Ante-mortem thrombi are frequently present in the left ventricle and occasionally in the right ventricle and atrium. The atria are also dilated. There is fibrous thickening of the endocardium and this is most prominent in the left ventricle. This is diffuse in some cases but tends to be more marked over some areas, particularly the apex of the left ventricle (Fig. 1.7).

Infarcts are present in about half the cases and are distributed amongst lungs, kidneys, spleen and brain. There is no evidence of any associated congenital heart lesion and the foramen ovale is closed in all cases. Histologically, when the fibrous thickening is mild to moderate, it is composed of both collagen and elastic, the latter being most prominent adjacent to the myocardium (Fig. 1.8). When the endocardial thickening is marked, collagen predominates. The thickened endocardium in most cases contains a sprinkling of lymphocytes and plasma cells with occasional neutrophils. The trabeculae carneae are often encased in fibrous tissue and the fibrous thickening usually

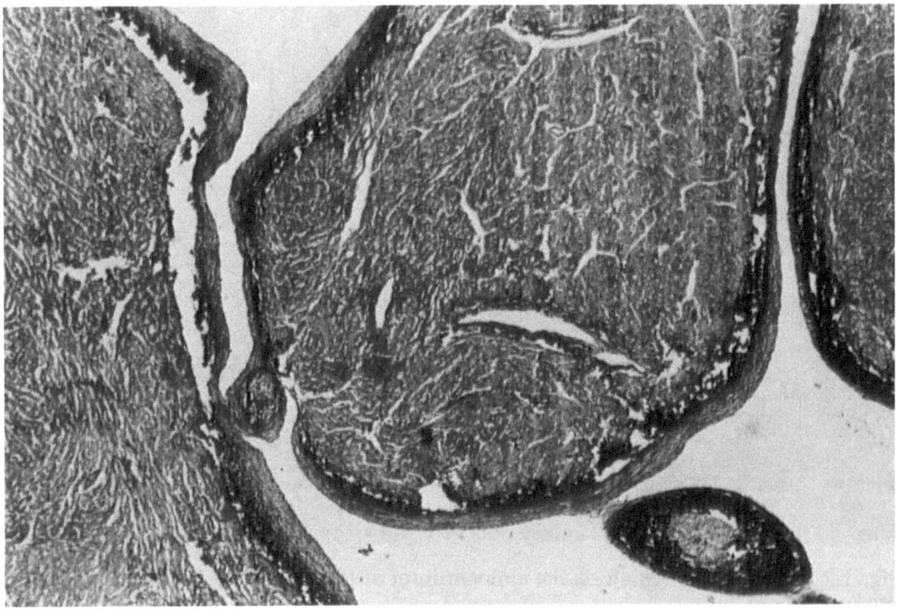

Fig. 1.8. Fibro-elastotic thickening of the endocardium of the papillary muscles. Elastic Masson, ×35

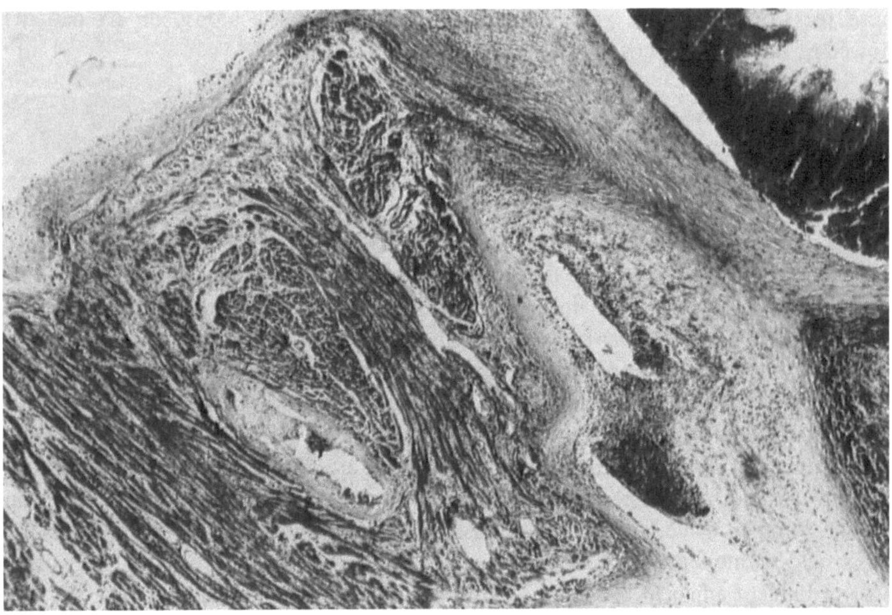

Fig. 1.9. Marked fibrous endocardial thickening with involvement of the Thebesian veins. Elastic-Masson, ×35

involves the Thebesian veins (Fig. 1.9). However, the fibrosis does not extend on to the valves in any instance. In areas where the endocardial thickening is not marked, there is often necrosis and fibrosis of the sub-endocardial muscle fibres. When patches of gross endocardial thickening are present these appear to be due to organization of intraluminal thrombi. In such instances the elastic in the fibrous tissue is confined to the part of the endocardium abutting on the myocardium. In the cases with more diffuse fibrous endocardial thickening, the thickening appears to be independent of thrombus formation. Thrombi, when present, are most prominent between the interstices of the trabeculae carneae.

The myocardial muscle fibres are hypertrophied and often show foci of interstitial fibrosis with occasional chronic inflammatory cells. In addition the myocardial fibres are often swollen by a non specific intracellular oedema. The coronary arteries are normal in all instances. Apart from infarction in some subjects, the remaining organs show the usual changes associated with congestive cardiac failure.

Pathogenesis of Idiopathic Cardiac Hypertrophy in Children

There are differences between these cases and the reports of infantile endocardial fibroelastosis. The latter condition is a disease of infancy usually presenting within the first six months of life or within the first year, whereas only three of the African cases presented below one year of age and none had associated congenital heart lesions. In addition none had valvular involvement secondary to the fibroelastosis. Clinically and pathologically, these cases appear to be very similar to those reported in adults in South Africa as idiopathic heart disease. It is however, unlikely, that aetiologically, they are similar.

There is no clinical evidence that nutritional factors are of importance, although the possibility of their being the sequelae of earlier kwashiorkor cannot entirely be excluded (*Smythe* et al. 1962). The most likely possibility is that these are examples of post viral myocarditis, although cases of viral myocarditis are not frequently diagnosed clinically, and rarely come to autopsy. It seems likely that the primary dysfunction is myocardial, the endocardial lesions being secondary. It has been suggested that many of the endocardial changes are a response to cardiac dilatation and that the sclerotic endocardium is a support rather than an impediment to myocardial function (*Black-Schaffer* 1957). An additional factor accounting for some of the endocardial changes is that of superimposed mural thrombosis. Organization of these thrombi produces marked endocardial fibrosis. This is usually seen where stasis is most likely i.e., in the apices of the ventricles and between the interstices of the trabeculae carneae. The endocardial thickening involves the arterioluminal and Thebesian veins and causes ischaemia of the inner third of the myocardium which is nourished from the lumen of the heart via these vessels.

Summary

Idiopathic cardiomyopathy is a common cause of heart failure in the Black population of South Africa. In approximately half the males the underlying aetiology is probably ethanol, but in the majority of the females, all the children and half the males ethanol can play no part in the pathogenesis. Although malnutrition probably plays some role, as yet no specific mechanism has been outlined. The effect on the adult heart of kwashiorkor in childhood is undetermined and warrants further investigation. There is no evidence to suggest a familial incidence.

Chapter 2

Hypertension and Coronary Artery Disease

Hyertension

Hypertension is very common in Blacks and occurs at a younger age than in Whites. It behaves in an explosive manner with death occurring frequently from cerebral haemorrhage, uraemia or congestive cardiac failure. In a study of urban Zulus, *Seedat* et al. (1978) found that the mean arterial pressure according to age and sex was not as high as in the American Negro, West Indian or Nigerian, but certainly higher than in most Caucasian populations. In the clinical series of *Schwartz* et al. (1958) hypertension was third in the frequency of cardiac disorders after idiopathic heart failure and chronic rheumatic heart disease and comprised 19.6% of all their cardiac cases. Recent authors have however, stressed that with increasing urbanization and associated stress, the incidence of hypertension in Blacks has increased and will probably rise even further. *Wyndham* (1979) has stated that the pattern of mortality from diseases of the circulatory system of Blacks in South Africa is that of high mortality rate for cerebral vascular disease and hypertensive heart disease and very low mortality rate for ischaemic heart disease. The current accepted view is that, in Johannesburg, the second most common cause of death in the adult Black population (after violence) is hypertension and its complications (*Seftel* 1973). There has been dispute as to whether hypertension in Blacks is essential or secondary to underlying renal disease. *Isaacson* and *Kincaid-Smith* (1962) examined the autopsy records of patients over the age of fifty years who had died of natural causes. Patients who had had a blood pressure of 200/100 mm Hg or more and had died of the effects of hypertension such as heart failure, uraemia or cerebral haemorrhage, were selected for study.

Sixty four per cent of the cases presented the features of essential nephrosclerosis and 36% had underlying renal disease. Only 10% of the total showed chronic pyelonephritis. A feature was the comparatively young age of the patients, 57% being between 30 and 49 years of age. The high incidence of malignant hypertension (48%) was also noteworthy. The incidence of chronic pyelonephritis in hypertensive Black subjects was thus lower than in a similar series from London (*Kincaid-Smith* et al. 1958). It is therefore apparent that essential hypertension is the final pathological diagnosis in most cases of severe hypertension in Blacks, and that renal disease plays an even less important role than in the White populations of South Africa or Britain. Similarly, in a renal biopsy study of pregnant hypertensive subjects, *Seftel* et al. (1960) showed that essential hypertension is by far the commonest pathological finding and that underlying renal disease, including pyelonephritis, is comparatively infrequent.

Recently *Isaacson* (1977) confirmed the high incidence of hypertensive heart disease at autopsy (see Tables 1.1, 1.2).

In Zimbabwe hypertension is one of the commonest diseases in the Black population, and in the resident population of Salisbury hypertension, (including cerebrovascular disease) accounts for 15% of the total deaths of Black adults over the age of 39 years (*Jones* et al. 1974). This percentage is very similar to the corresponding figure of 16% of Whites and is in striking contrast to ischaemic heart disease which kills 27% of Whites compared with 2% of Black adults over the age of 39 years. *Seedat* and *Reddy* (1974) in Durban found accelerated hypertension clinically in 7% of their Black hypertensives with death occurring frequently in uraemia.

They too found that ischaemic heart disease was very infrequent in Black hypertensives, in contrast to Indian hypertensives who manifested ischaemic heart disease in 12% of cases. The rarity of ischaemic heart disease in hypertensives suggests that in Blacks hypertension is not that important a predisposing factor to myocardial infarction.

In contrast to the findings in Southern Africa, *Shaper* (1972) reporting from Uganda found that glomerulo nephritis was present in 42% of his subjects, accounting for nearly all cases of hypertensive heart disease, at necropsy under the age of 30 years. He suggested that chronic renal disease, particularly glomerulonephritis, is an important cause of severe and fatal hypertension in young people in tropical countries. His findings received support from *Hutt* and *Coles* (1969) also from Uganda who claimed that glomerulonephritis was the underlying disorder in one third of hypertensive subjects coming to postmortem, and accounted for nearly all cases of hypertension at necropsy under the age of thirty. Hypertension in either sex under 40 years of age in Uganda is likely to be secondary to renal disease, usually glomerulonephritis. In older patients essential hypertension is common and seen more frequently in males. In Nigeria however, *Akingkugbe* (1969) found that of 210 cases of hypertension seen over a three year period, essential hypertension accounted for the majority. However, in hypertensive Nigerian children, glomerulonephritis is the most frequent finding (*Aderele* and *Seriki* 1974).

Coronary Artery Disease

Introduction

Many authors have shown that the severity of atherosclerosis is considerably less in Blacks than in corresponding White subjects (*Becker* 1946; *Higginson* and *Pepler* 1954; *Sacks* 1960; *Wainwright* 1961). The comparative infrequency of severe coronary atherosclerosis is parallelled by the rarity of myocardial infarction (*Becker* 1946; *Brock* and *Bronte-Stewart* 1955; *Bronte-Stewart* et al. 1955; *Schrire* and *Uys* 1958; *Schrire* 1961; *Reef* and *Isaacson* 1962; *Seedat* and *Pillay* 1977). An occasional Black may show severe atheroma as severe as in the White, but there are many aortas from elderly Africans which are almost free of atheroma. In the aorta the thick spongy atheromatous plaques which readily ulcerate are rare in the Black, as are the completely calcified rigid coronary arteries so common in elderly Whites (*Wainwright* 1961). Atherosclerotic aneurysms are similarly infrequent, although cerebral softening does not show the same low incidence. Claims that the rarity of myocardial infarction in Blacks is due to a specific pattern of coronary artery distribution in the black heart (*Brink* 1949), have been completely refuted (*Singer* 1959).

In comparing South African Blacks with the New Orleans Negro and White man in the same age group, *Strong* et al. (1959) found fatty streaks to be present universally in all three groups to some extent after the first decade, but showed that the prevalence and quantitative extent of fibrous plaques were however considerably less in the South African Blacks than in the other two groups, and they suggested that the development of fibrous plaques might be related to the process of fibrin deposition and organization or vascularization within fatty streaks, a view that received some support from the high levels of fibrinolysis observed in Blacks (*Gillman* et al. 1957) and with the more rapid development of fibrinolysis (*Mersky* et al. 1958).

Anderson et al. (1959) felt that the differences in the severity of atherosclerosis were insufficient to explain the markedly different incidence in myocardial infarction and coronary occlusion in Black and White subjects. The disparity in Blacks between occasionally severe atherosclerosis of the aorta and the low mortality from coronary occlusion has been noted by several authors (*Walker* and *Simson* 1958; *Sacks* 1960).

Reef and *Isaacson* (1962) undertook a study of the degree of atherosclerosis of every artery in a series of 32 consecutive autopsies in subjects over 50 years old. As cerebrovascular accidents, particularly haemorrhage, are not infrequent in Blacks, it was expected that atherosclerosis would be more severe in the cerebral vessels as compared with the coronary arteries, but contrary to expectations, the cerebral vessels showed less atheroma than did the coronary arteries, and in addition, atheroma in one artery did not necessarily reflect the degree of atheroma in another artery in the same subject. The peripheral vessels never showed significant atheroma.

The above observations have been correlated by most authors with the low fat content of the diet of the South African Black and the associated low mean and serum cholesterol (*Brock* and *Bronte-Stewart* 1955; *Bronte-Stewart* et al. 1955).

Myocardial infarction is rare not only in South African Blacks, but in the indigenous populations throughout Africa (*Williams* 1969; *Koate* et al. 1971; *Williams* et al. 1971; *Bertrand* et al. 1974).

With increasing urbanization and westernization of the Black people of South Africa, an alteration in the distribution of the various types of cardiac disease would be expected both clinically and at necropsy. To investigate this possibility, the post-mortem records at Baragwanath Hospital for 1959 and 1960 were compared with those for 1976. Baragwanath Hospital is a large (2500 bed) hospital for Blacks which supplies the medical services for the town of Soweto on the outskirts of Johannesburg. The precise population of Soweto is uncertain but estimates vary between 900 000 and 1.2 million. The population has increased gradually over the years and there has been a concomitant rise in the standard of living; there is now a small, but nevertheless significant, fairly affluent middle class composed of professionals, including teachers and doctors, businessmen and better-paid white collar workers in sedentary occupations. The process of industrialization, urbanization and westernization has been accelerated in recent years.

Material and Methods

All the autopsy records for 1959, 1960 and 1976 were extracted and the deaths from cardiac disease examined in detail. The deaths from cardiac disease were expressed as a percentage of the total autopsies for that year, and in addition each category of cardiac disease was expressed as a percentage of the total number of autopsies done on cardiac patients. While this may not be an accurate reflection of the true incidence of the various types of cardiac disease in this population, it does however give an approximation.

Results

The striking finding is the marked increase in the percentage of cases of myocardial infarction (see Table 1.1). Of the 14 cases in 1976, 10 showed coronary artery occlusion and 4 showed marked narrowing of the coronary arteries with interstitial fibrosis and heart failure from myocardial ischaemia. The figure for 1976 is 2.0% of all autopsies compared with 0.13% in both 1959 and 1960. Expressed as a percentage of the total number of necropsies done on cardiac patients, cases of myocardial infarction have increased from 0.9% in 1959 and 0.81% in 1960 to 11.7% in 1976.

Discussion

In 1959 and 1960 myocardial infarction comprised less than 1% of all cardiac deaths found at necropsy, whereas in 1976 it comprised 11.7%, a thirteenfold increase in incidence. Nevertheless, the incidence of myocardial infarction is still very low in this population. *Walker* (1969, 1974) has stated that the equivalent White population would have about 700 cases per annum of myocardial infarction and sudden death. Although *Seftel* and *Kew* (1970) have shown that coronary heart disease is still uncommon in the Johannesburg Black it is on the other hand not so rare, that it can continue to be largely ignored in differential diagnosis. Nevertheless, in a recent study *Seedat* and *Pillay* (1977) have shown that one of the striking features at autopsy among hypertensive Black patients is the rarity of myocardial infarction and the frequent occurrence of congestive cardiac failure and cerebrovascular accident as a result of hypertension. A ten year post mortem study among 434 African patients suffering from hypertension showed that only 2.2% had myocardial infarction. The increase of coronary heart disease within the last 20 years is less than would be expected and despite the increasing measure of sophistication of diet and manner of life, the Blacks of South Africa have possibly the lowest coronary heart disease mortality of any intensively urbanized population in the world.

The low mortality is suprising since data on weight indicate that many are overweight, hypertension is very common and their physical activity, although greater than Whites, is decreasing every day in proportion to level of prosperity. Smoking is prevalent. The rarity of coronary heart disease may be due to a racial factor or due to environmental factors such as the comparatively low proportion of heavy smokers. *Seftel*

(1978) concluded that the rarity of coronary heart disease in Blacks is not enigmatic, but is appropriate to their environmental circumstances. He assessed various risk factors including affluence, age, hypertension, hyperlipidaemia, dietary excess, smoking, physical inactivity, diabetes, obesity, hyperuricaemia and hyperinsulinism and concluded that among males only hypertension, and among females only hypertension and obesity emerged as prominent factors, and neither of these is significantly atherogenic in the social, nutritional and metabolic milieu in which Blacks generally live.

The rise in incidence over the 16 year period is nevertheless of significance, and must be ascribed to the increasing level of prosperity being enjoyed by a significant class of Blacks, who can now consume meat containing large quantitites of fat, smoke heavily, and travel in limousines. In an African developing population in which diseases consequent on an increasing severity of atherosclerosis are considered, the first to emerge is cerebrovascular disease followed by coronary heart disease and finally peripheral vascular disease (*Walker* 1975). Coronary heart disease has been shown to be uncommon in Blacks in contrast to its frequency and severity in many Caucasian groups, but cerebral atheroma and the resulting complications have been much less closely examined. While South African Blacks seem to have less coronary and aortic atheroma thus producing little clinical disease compared with Whites, the Black cerebral vessels are a mystery, as clinical cerebrovascular occlusive disease is supposedly commoner than coronary occlusive disease. However, these findings have never been confirmed pathologically, and there are many difficulties in the way of establishing accurate statistics. Subjects with cerebral infarcts are much less likely to die and therefore come to autopsy than those with cerebral haemorrhage, and in addition, should they die there is much more likelihood of their dying at home than in hospital (*Isaacson* 1978).

Summary

Hypertension is common amongst Blacks and is in the majority of instances of the essential type. Despite the high incidence of hypertension, coronary heart disease is rare, although with increasing westernization and urbanization there has been a slight but significant rise in the number of cases seen at autopsy. The low incidence of myocardial infarction is probably attributable to the absence of factors other than hypertension generally associated with atherosclerosis in westernized subjects. There is a disparity between the occasionally severe atherosclerosis of the aorta and the low mortality for coronary occlusion.

Chapter 3

Rheumatic Heart Disease, Aortitis, Miscellaneous Cardiovascular Diseases

Rheumatic Heart Disease

There is overwhelming evidence that rheumatic heart disease is today the commonest form of heart disease in children and young adults in most tropical or developing countries, and one of the most common cardiovascular diseases in adults (*Shaper* 1972). Not only is it common but there is clinical and necropsy evidence from several countries that the frequency of the disease is increasing. In almost all tropical studies on acute rheumatic fever, the proportion of very young children affected is regarded as higher than in temperate climates. In Johannesburg, when African children were compared with American and British children, the African group showed twice the percentage of children under five years of age (*Chesler* et al. 1966) and many children under ten years of age have severe valvular disease. Thus, tropical rheumatic fever affects the younger age group, and the severity, as measured by early mortality, is greater than in temperate countries. Acute rheumatic fever exists in a virulent form in Blacks because of the youth of the patients and the frequency of carditis and congestive cardiac failure, and a higher proportion of deaths in the younger age groups (*Schrire* 1958; *Chesler* et al. 1966). *Schwartz* et al. (1958) showed that acute and chronic rheumatic heart disease accounted for 23.3% of the cases of heart disease admitted to one of the medical wards at Baragwanath Hospital and was second in frequency only to idiopathic cardiomyopathy. The high incidence of rheumatic heart disease in Blacks can be equated with a high prevalence of streptococcal infection and its consequences, which are among the many schedules of poverty, one of the many afflictions that can be rooted out by socio-economic amelioration (*Spodick* 1975). In the necropsy series of *Higginson* et al. (1960) rheumatic heart disease accounted for 32.5% of all cardiac deaths and was thus the commonest cardiac disease at postmortem.

In the Blacks of South Africa acute rheumatic carditis is seen in a virulent form comparable to what was seen in the White population of Britain 50 years ago. Young patients dying of acute diffuse rheumatic carditis before the development of chronic valvular lesions are not infrequently seen. Instances occur of extension of the rheumatic process onto the adjacent aorta with the development of a severe diffuse aortitis.

Not infrequently patients develop severe congestivecardiac failure during an episode of acute rheumatic fever and emergency prosthetic surgery may be necessary.

In a large autopsy series referred to previously (*Isaacson* 1977), rheumatic heart disease comprised 3.1% of all autopsies in 1959, 4.3% in 1960 and 3.6% in 1976, and an average of 23.3% of all necropsies on cardiac patients (see Tables 1.1, 1.2). The total number of necropsied cases for the years 1959, 1960 and 1976 was 80, of whom 45 were female and 35 male; 61% were below the age of 39 years. The distribution of

Table 3.1. Distribution of valvular lesions in chronic rheumatic heart disease (*Isaacson* 1977)

Shaper et al. (1968)			Current series		
Decimal-ized fraction[a]	Lesion	Number	Decimal-ized fraction[a]	Lesion	Number
	Mitral valve alone	99		Mitral valve alone	36
0.58	Mitral and aortic valves	57	0.53	Mitral and aortic valves	19
0.25	Aortic valve alone	25	0.25	Aortic valve alone	9
0.18	Mitral and tricuspid valves	18	0.19	Mitral and tricuspid valves	7
0.12	Mitral tricuspid and aortic valves	12	0.08	Mitral, tricuspid and aortic valves	3
	Mitral and pulmonary valves	1		Mitral and pulmonary valves	–
	Mitral, tricuspid and pulmonary valves	1		Mitral, tricuspid and pulmonary valves	–

[a] See text for explanation

the valvular lesions in a necropsy study from Uganda (*Shaper* et al. 1968) is shown in Table 3.1. The Ugandan findings were compared with the present series. The number of patients who had mitral valvular disease alone was used as the denominator of a fraction and the other lesions were used respectively as the numerator, the subsequent fraction then being expressed as a decimal. The Ugandan findings were almost identical with those of the current series.

The recent advances in cardiac surgery do not appear to have significantly reduced the incidence of chronic rheumatic heart disease at autopsy. This is not a reflection on the efficacy of cardiac surgery but indicates that the number of cases coming to surgery represents the tip of an iceberg.

Idiopathic Aortitis

This condition was first reported by *Isaacson* et al. (1959) who described two cases in African children. The one, a female of nine years was admitted in congestive cardiac failure with a raised blood pressure in the upper limbs, and a diagnosis of coarctation of the aorta with left ventricular enlargement. Before operation could be performed, she died, and at autopsy a large thrombus partially occluded the aorta from 6 cm distal to the origin of the left subclavian artery to 2.5 cm proximal to the origin of the coeliac artery. The second case was that of an eight year old female who presented in congestive cardiac failure with hypertension, and at autopsy showed renal artery thrombosis as a result of extension of the aortic arteritis to the renal artery. In 1961 *Isaacson* reported six cases of this condition calling it an "Idiopathic aortitis in young Africans". The ages of the patients varied from seven to sixteen years; there were two males and four females. Nearly all the cases showed a sustained and constant elevation

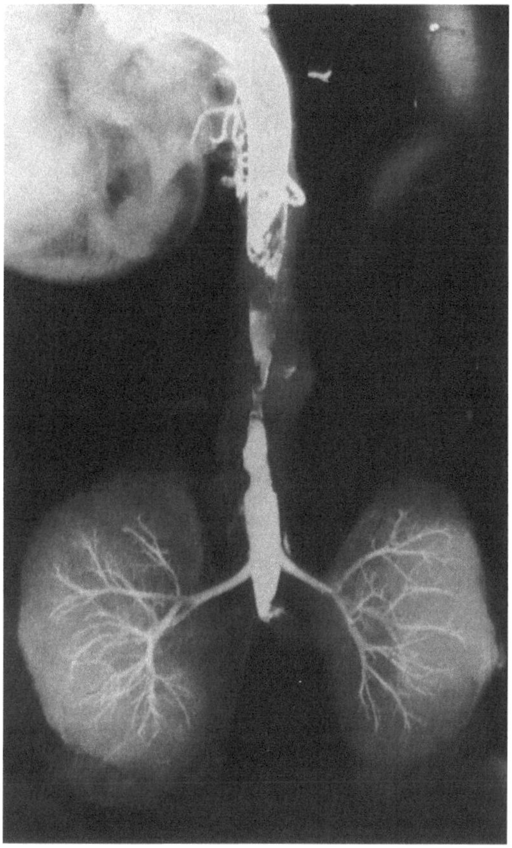

Fig. 3.1. Post mortem radiograph demonstrating narrowing of the thoracic and abdominal aorta with shrinkage of one kidney due to partial occlusion of the renal artery

in blood pressure, in most instances due to renal artery obstruction. Pathologically, the condition resembled Takayasu's arteritis.

Pathology

Virtually any part of the aorta may be affected. Most cases show involvement of the abdominal aorta with occlusion of one renal artery producing hypertension. The aorta shows areas of dilatation alternating with foci of narrowing. There are areas of considerable thickening of the aortic wall and foci of superimposed intimal thrombosis. In many instances the thrombotic process extends to involve one or other of the renal arteries (Figs. 3.1–3.5). Microscopically, the lumen of the aorta is often markedly narrowed by both old fibrous intimal thickening and recent antemortem thrombus. The adventitia is fibrosed and shows heavy focal infiltration by plasma cells and lymphocytes.

In some areas the inflammatory cells may extend into the media for a short distance and here the elastic is fragmented and frayed. In parts, the entire wall of the aorta may appear to have disintegrated and to have become incorporated in the throm-

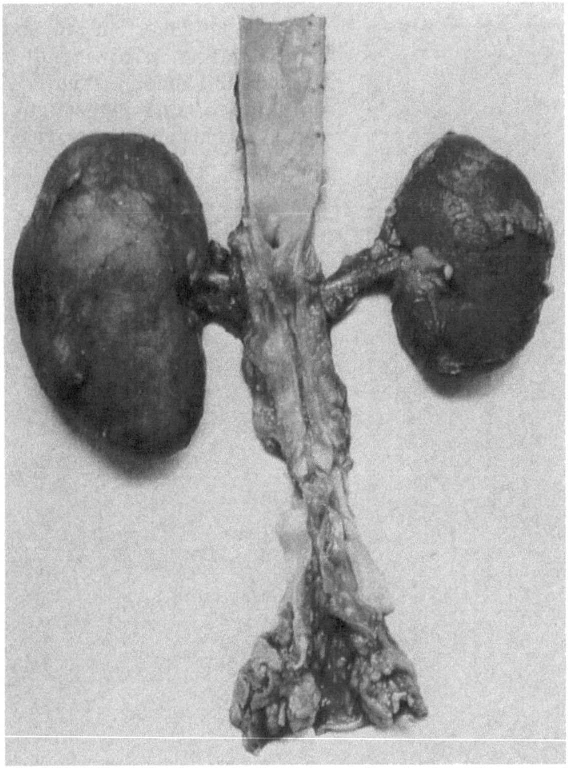

Fig. 3.2. Shrinkage of one kidney due to partial occlusion of the renal artery. The aorta below the origin of the renal arteries shows marked narrowing of the lumen with considerable fibrous thickening of the wall

bus. The wall is heavily infiltrated by chronic inflammatory cells and many of the vasa vasorum show endarteritis. In the most severely affected parts of the aorta there is replacement fibrosis of the elastic and muscle by dense accellular collagen (Figs. 3.6–3.9).

In the presence of hypertension, the heart shows left ventricular hypertrophy and the remaining organs show passive venous congestion if congestive cardiac failure has been present. In an occasional case the para aortic lymph nodes have been found to show a granulomatous reaction resembling tuberculosis, and it has been suggested that a hypersensitivity reaction to the tubercle bacillus in the para aortic lymph nodes may set up a reactive endarteritis of the vasa vasorum (*Isaacson* and *Shnier* 1961).

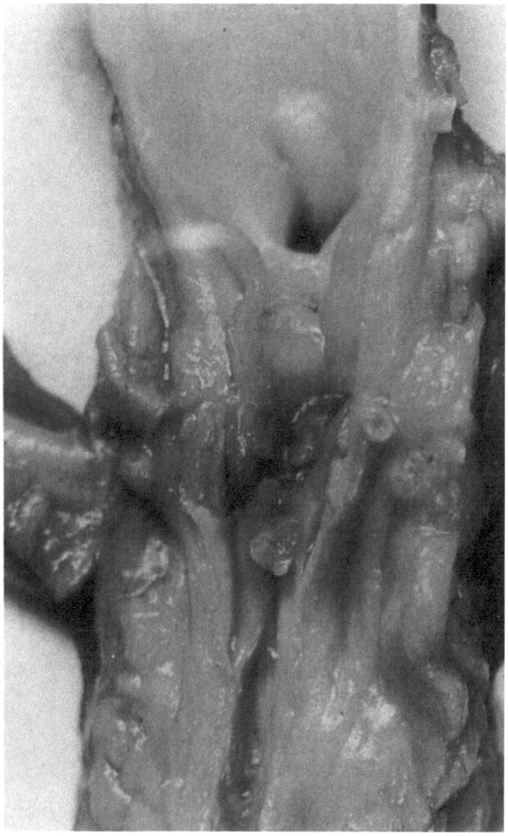

Fig. 3.3. Marked narrowing of the lumen of the aorta with considerable fibrous thickening of the wall

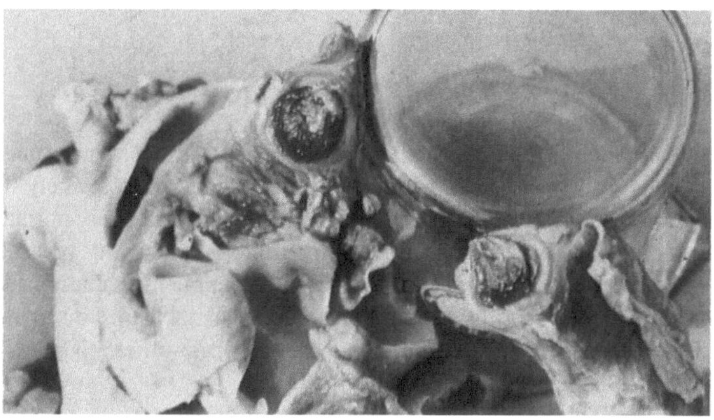

Fig. 3.4. Occlusion of the aorta beyond the origin of the subclavian artery

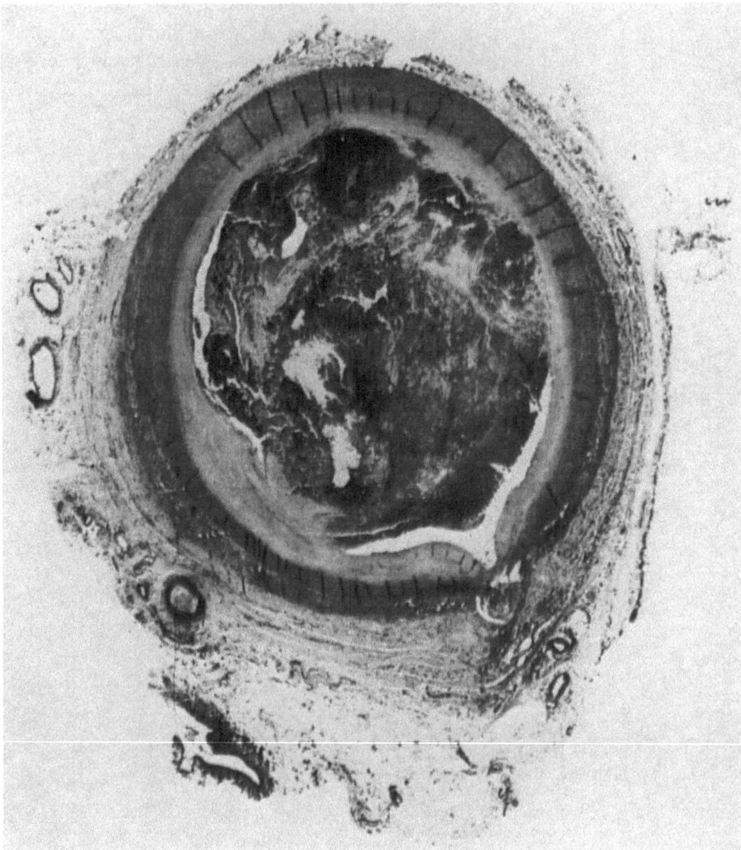

Fig. 3.5. Occluded thoracic aorta. Note the marked intimal thickening and the occlusion of the vasa vasorum. H%E, × 10

Differentiation from Other Forms of Aortitis

Syphilis

Syphilis can generally be excluded serologically. Syphilitic aortitis does not usually extend below the diaphragm and generally affects the ascending aorta most severely. In cases of idiopathic aortitis the ascending aorta is not infrequently completely normal. Aortitis due to acquired syphilis at the early age at which idiopathic aortitis presents can be excluded, as the average time between infection with treponema pallidum and the development of symptoms of aortitis is twenty years, the peak incidence occurring between forty and fifty years. If congenital syphilis were the cause other stigmata of the disease would have been present.

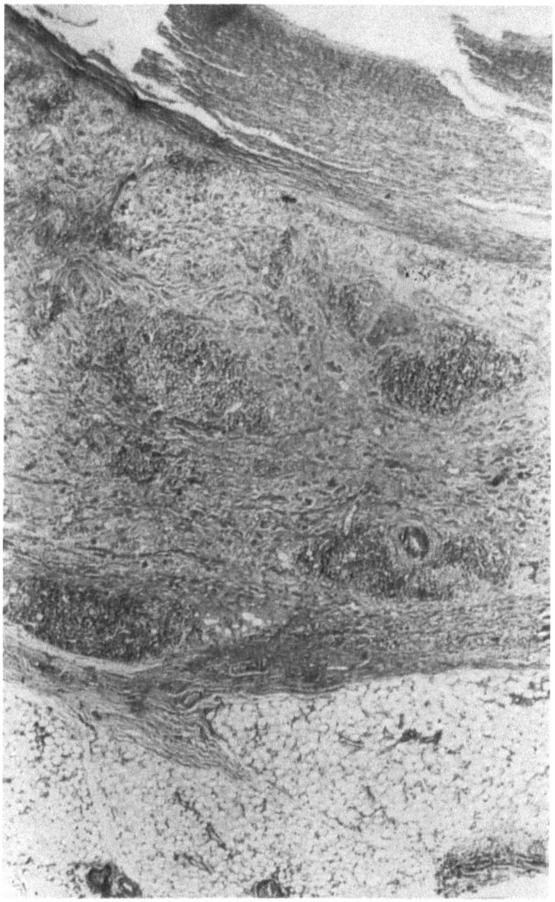

Fig. 3.6. Heavy inflammatory infiltrate around the vasa vasorum with marked fibrous thickening of the adventitia of the aorta. H&E, ×23

Fig. 3.7. Clumping and destruction of the elastica in the media. Elastic-Masson, ×95
▼

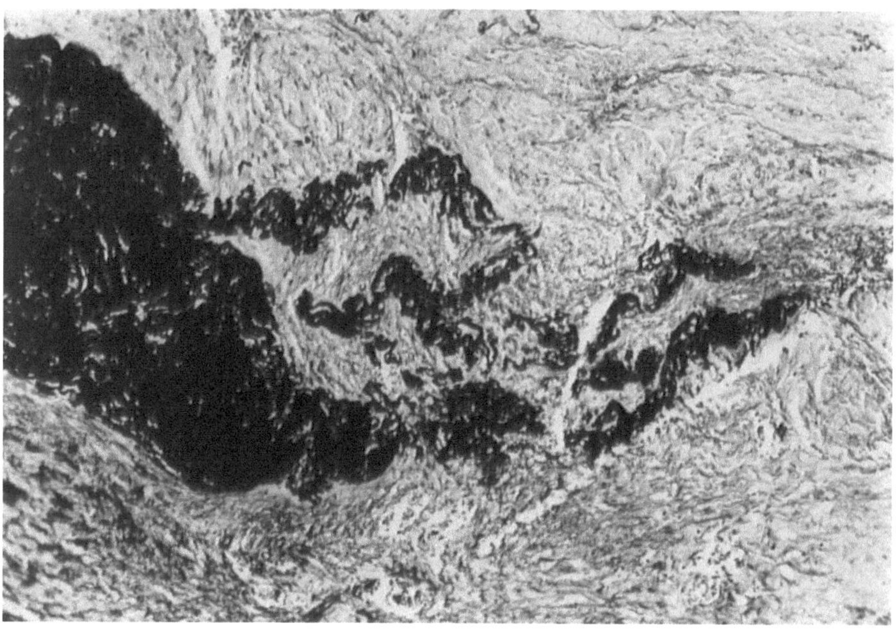

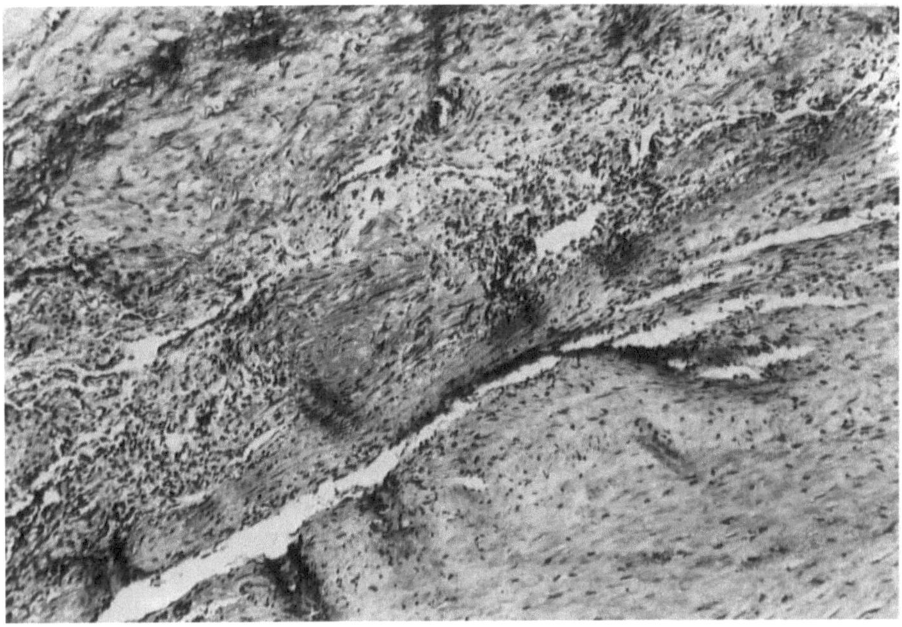

▲ **Fig. 3.8.** Marked fibrous intimal thickening with a diffuse infiltrate of inflammatory cells in the media. H&E, ×100

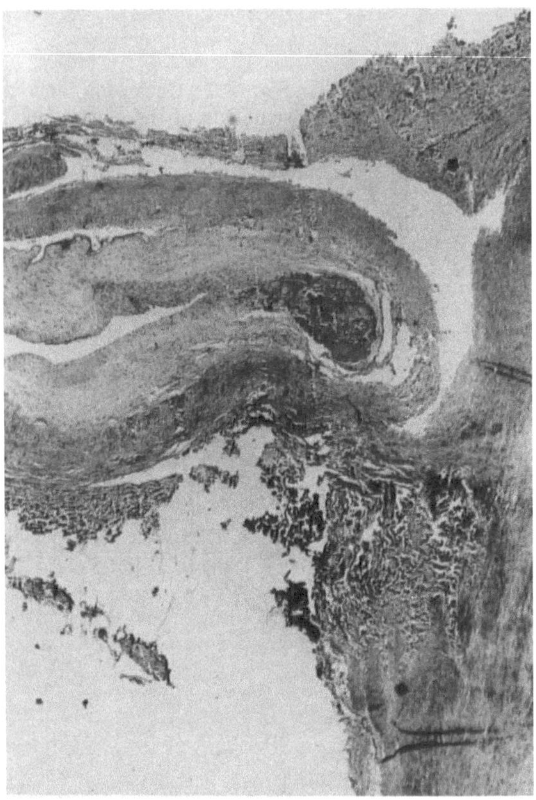

Fig. 3.9. Occluded renal artery with intimal fibrous thickening. H&E, ×30

Takayasu's Arteritis

Initially, it was thought that the arteritic process was limited to the aortic arch and its branches, but recent studies (*Ueno* et al. 1967; *Lupi-Herrera* et al. 1977) have defined three varieties of the disease, affecting respectively the aortic arch and its branches only, the thoracic descending aorta and the abdominal aorta, and the third type showing involvement of the descending aorta, the abdominal aorta and the arch. *Lupi-Herrera* et al. (1977) have suggested a fourth type with involvement of the pulmonary artery. The majority of subjects are females and in 77% the age of onset is between 10 and 20 years. In 65% of cases the aortic trunks and abdominal aorta are involved. Forty eight percent give a previous history of tuberculosis. Clinically and pathologically idiopathic aortitis is indistinguishable from Takayasu's arteritis.

Giant Cell Arteritis

Giant cell arteritis involves medium sized muscular arteries in most instances, although involvement of the aorta is not unknown (*Cardell* and *Hanley* 1951). It usually occurs in elderly subjects. The histological picture is characterised by large numbers of giant cells, which probably arise in a reaction to degenerating elastic tissue.

Miscellaneous Forms of Aortitis

Rheumatoid arthritis, rheumatic fever and tuberculosis may cause aortitis but none of the patients showed any of the features of these diseases. The possible relationship to tuberculosis has already been mentioned.

In one instance of idiopathic aortitis presenting with hypertension and an abnormal aortogram radiologically, the patient developed an uncontrollable episode of hypertensive encephalopathy immediately after undergoing skin testing for tuberculosis. The skin test was repeated and on each occasion produced an immediate attack of hypertensive encephalopathy.

Aetiology of Idiopathic Aortitis

No infective agent was isolated and no history was ever obtained of administration of witch-doctor medicines. The possible relationship to tuberculosis has already been discussed.

Myxoid Degeneration of Heart Valves

This condition affects mainly the mitral valve and is characterized by transformation of the normally dense cusp fibrosa into a loose metachromatically staining connective tissue (*Pomerance* and *Davies* 1975). The valve leaflet stretches and results in a large "floppy" cusp which prolapses into the atrium in systole. Clinically, this is the same condition that has been described as the billowing mitral valve leaflet (*Barlow* and *Bosman* 1966; *Bittar* and *Sosa* 1968; *Frable* 1969; *Pocock* and *Barlow* 1971).

Usually the mitral valve is affected almost exclusively, the posterior cusp being affected more often and more severely than the anterior resulting in a marked increase in the surface area of the affected cusp. Occasionally similar changes can be seen in the tricuspid valve but the aortic valve is very rarely affected. The microscopic picture shows loose spongy metachromatic acid mucopolysaccharide replacing the normal dense collagen. No inflammatory cell infiltration or increased fibrosis is found. Similar changes may be seen in the chordae tendineae.

The condition is not infrequent in the urban Black although the precise incidence has not yet been ascertained (*Isaacson* 1980). This could only be done following a complete re-evaluation of the histological sections of all "rheumatic valves" removed at surgery over a period of years.

In a small series of nine cases there were four males and five females. The ages varied from 21 years to 66 years, five being under 40 years of age and two under 25 years of age. In six, the aortic valves were affected and in only three were the mitral valves involved. In all other studies the condition has affected mainly the mitral valve (*Pomerance* 1969), and has been reported as uncommon below the age of fifty years. In this small series five of the nine cases were under the age of 40 years and two were under 25 years of age.

The predominance of aortic valve involvement is of interest in relation to the study by *Pepler* (1955) who, in a series of unselected 144 aortas in Black subjects found increased metachromatic material in practically every case. Severe cystic medial degeneration was present in 17 of the 144 cases. It may very well be that mucoid degenerative changes including myxomatous degeneration of the cardiac valves is more frequent in Blacks than in Whites.

Intimomedial Mucoid Degeneration

Decker et al. (1977) reported 9 unusual cases of abdominal aortic aneurysms. They occurred in a younger age group than atherosclerotic aneurysms and with a female predominance. The ages ranged from 39 to 64 years with a mean of 51.1 years. There were 7 females and 2 males. More than half the patients had hypertension and three presented with severe abdominal pain due to rupture of the aneurysm. Serological tests for syphilis were negative.

The abdominal aorta alone was involved in six patients and in two the aneurysm involved both the aorta and the common iliac arteries. The aneurysms were below the level of the renal arteries in all cases, and in three subjects had ruptured retroperitoneally.

Macroscopically, these cases show a pale, almost white intimal surface with no evidence of fatty streaking or atheroma (Fig. 3.10). The adventitia is normal and the aneurysms can usually be excised with ease due to a notable lack of adventitial fibrosis and non-adherence of the vena cava. The histological changes in the aneurysms are characterized by mucoid thickening of the intima and attenuation of the media which

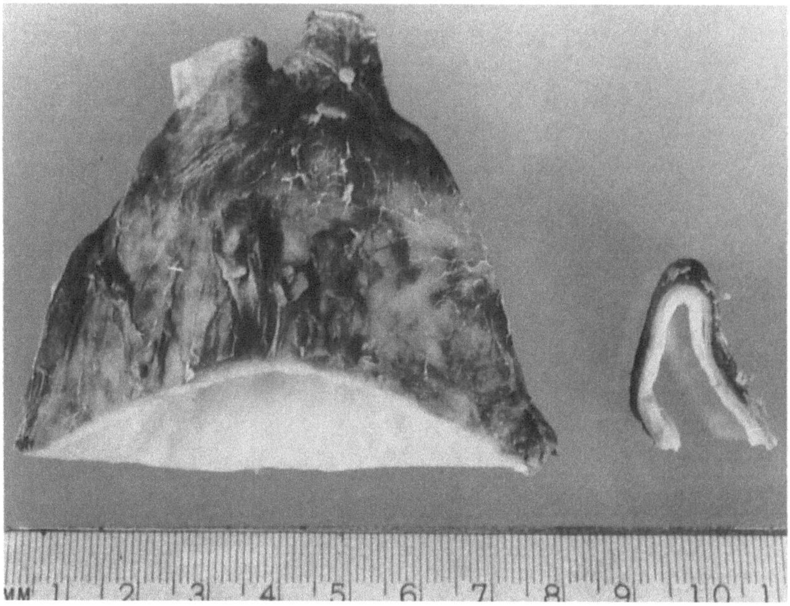

Fig. 3.10. Abdominal aneurysm from case of intimo medial mucoid degeneration. The intima is smooth and glistening and shows no evidence of atherosclerosis

is partially replaced by loose fibrous tissue. Large quantities of acid mucopolysaccharide are present in the media and intima. Splitting and fraying of the internal elastic lamina is present and in some areas the elastic tissue has completely disappeared. The absence of lipids and calcium in the media is striking. No inflammatory reaction is present (Figs. 3.11–3.13).

The changes do not resemble idiopathic aortitis. It may well be that in this population there is a spectrum of mucoid degeneration extending from the changes described in the aorta by *Pepler* (1955) to myxomatous degeneration of the heart valves and aneurysm formation in the aorta associated with intimomedial mucoid degeneration. None of the subjects show any of the features of Marfan's syndrome.

Miscellaneous

Idiopathic Mitral Subannular Left Ventricular Aneurysms

In 1962 *Abrahams* et al. described an unusual form of left ventricular aneurysm in Blacks which they termed annular subvalvar ventricular aneurysm. The aetiology was unknown, but congenital factors were considered important. The occurrence of this condition in Blacks living in such diverse environments as East and West Equatorial Africa, South Africa, West Indies and the United States suggests a genetic factor rather than any bacterial, viral, parasitic or dietetic aetiology (*Cockshott* et al. 1967). *Abra-*

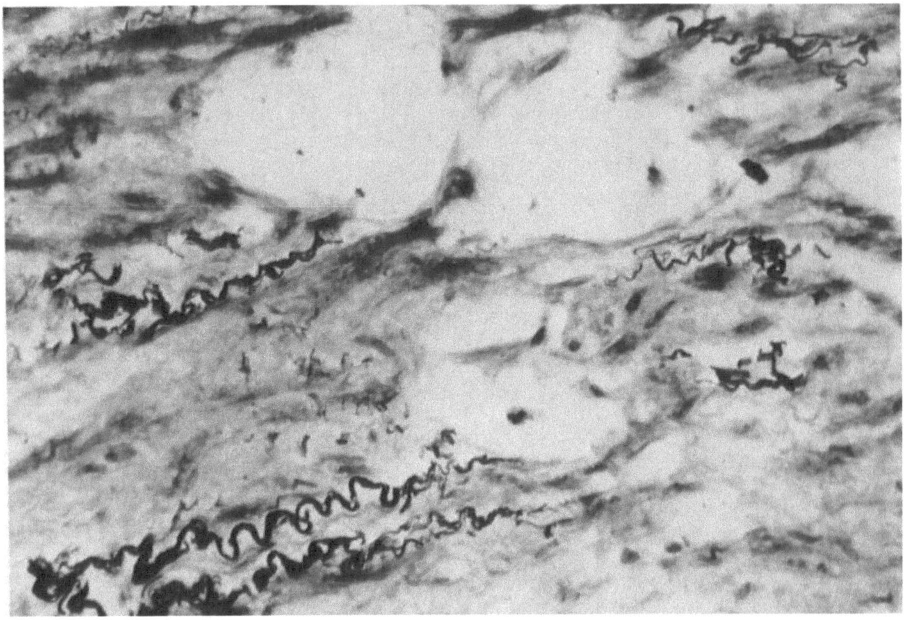

Fig. 3.11. Note cystic change in media with mucoid degeneration and disappearance of elastic tissue. Elastic-Masson, × 190

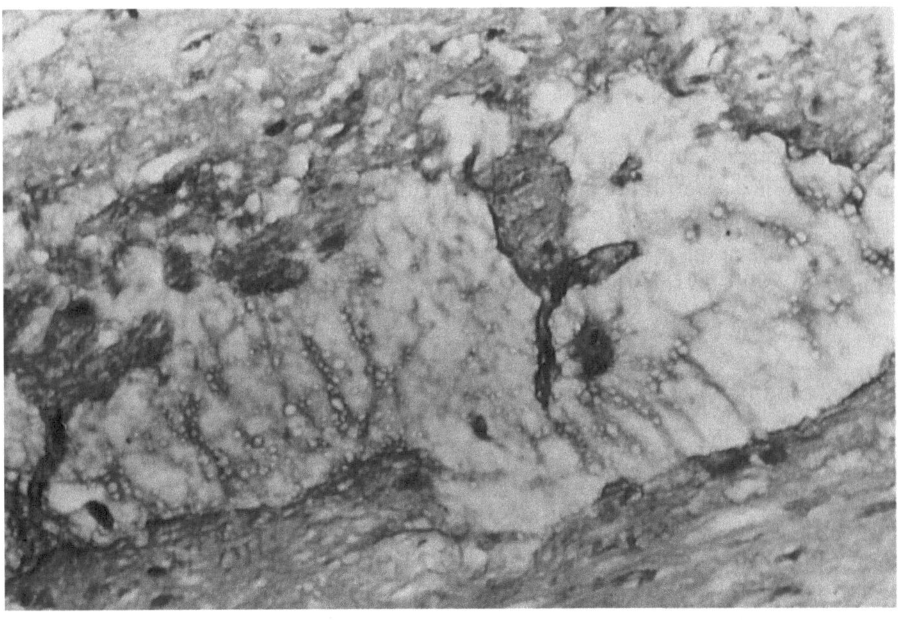

Fig. 3.12. Aneurysm wall showing area of mucoid change. Toluidine blue, × 180. Figures 3.12 and 3.13 are by courtesy of Professor *A. Schmaman*

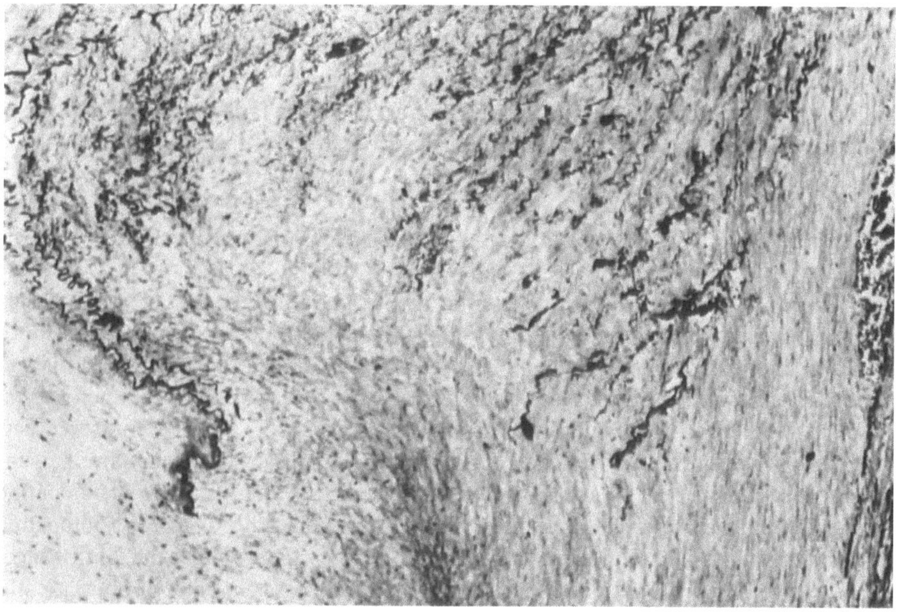

Fig. 3.13. Note loss of elastic tissue with evidence of thickened intima on the left. Elastic Masson, × 34

hams et al. (1962) considered the lesion a dissection or herniation of the left ventricle through a point of weakness where the myocardium is attached to the fibrous skeleton of the heart. The first such case from South Africa was that of a young Black woman aged 19 years dying of acute cardiac failure (*Higginson* and *Keeley* 1951). At autopsy, the heart showed a thin walled sac arising from the region of the mitral ring on the postero-lateral surface. This sac communicated with the left ventricle by an opening lateral to the mitral valve. Subsequently similar cases were reported from Durban (*Lurie* 1960) and Cape Town (*Becker* and *Schrire* 1969).

Most authors favour the view that the lesion is a congenital defect (*Robertson* and *Jackson* 1960). The condition is rare.

Cor Pulmonale

Kallichurum (1969) maintained that, in contrast to the generally accepted view, pulmonary thrombo-embolic disease with right ventricular strain and failure is a relatively common cause of cor pulmonale in Black subjects. She found thrombo-embolic cor pulmonale to be the second most common cause after fibrosing lung disease, of cor pulmonale in Blacks at postmortem. *Baker* and *Houlder* (1973) however, claimed that deep vein thrombosis in Black and Indian patients is lower than that reported in Whites and this is an accord with the observations in Zimbabwe (*Gelfand* and *Ross* 1976). However, *Joffey* (1974) maintained that White, Coloured, Black and Indian patients are all at a similar risk of post operative deep vein thrombosis.

In Uganda pulmonary thrombo-embolism has apparently become three times more frequent in the space of 21 years (*Drury* and *Mylius* 1973) and this has been ascribed to the increased consumption of sugar and fat.

In the Black population seen at Baragwanath Hospital fatal pulmonary embolism is a frequent finding at autopsy although incidence figures are unavailable.

The Changing Pattern of Heart Disease in South African Blacks

With increasing urbanization and Westernization of the Black people of South Africa a change is taking place in the distribution of the various types of cardiac disease both clinically and at necropsy (*Isaacson* 1977). Although still infrequent myocardial infarction has risen in incidence (see Tables 1.1, 1.2). Hypertension is common (*Seftel* 1973) and is increasing steadily in frequency (see Tables 1.1, 1.2). Seventyseven percent of hypertensives coming to necropsy are of the essential type. Fourtyfive percent are between the ages of 20 and 49 at the time of death. The incidence of idiopathic cardiomyopathy appears to have fallen. The male:female ratio of cases of idiopathic cardiomyopathy is 2:1. The condition starts as early as the third decade, but its highest incidence is from the fourth decade onwards. The cases in children must clearly have a different aetiology and pathogenesis from adults.

The incidence of rheumatic heart disease has not changed. Cor pulmonale and syphilitic aortitis comprise a very small percentage of cardiac deaths. There is a striking fall in the incidence of syphilitic aortitis which comprised 6.1% of all cardiac postmortems in the series of *Higginson* et al. (1960), 2.7% of all cardiac postmortems in 1959, 1.6% in 1960 and none in 1976.

Summary

Rheumatic heart disease is the commonest form of heart disease in children and young adults in this population. Idiopathic aortitis is a comparatively rare condition occurring in young Black subjects and is clinically and pathologically similar to Takayasu's syndrome. Intimomedial mucoid degeneration is different from Takayasu's arteritis and shows changes resembling those observed in Marfan's syndrome, although none of the patients have any of the stigmata of this syndrome. Myxoid degeneration of the heart valves (Barlow' syndrome) occurs not infrequently. The site of the lesion is different from that generally described in that the aortic valve is more frequently affected than the mitral. In addition the patients are younger than in other series. Idiopathic mitral subannular left ventricular aneurysms are rare and resemble those described in the rest of Africa. Cor pulmonale is not infrequent although the precise incidence is not known. The pattern of heart disease in South African Blacks is changing. There has been a rise in the incidence of myocardial infarction, a rise in the percentage of hypertensives and a fall in the number of cases with cardiomyopathy. There has been a marked drop in the incidence of syphilitic cardiovascular disease.

Chapter 4

Iron Overload

Iron overload of varying degree has been described in the Blacks of South Africa, Ghana, Malawi, Mozambique, Rhodesia and Tanzania. The greatest incidence occurs in the Blacks of Southern Africa where the majority of adults show varying degrees of tissue siderosis. Iron overload in Blacks is present throughout South Africa and estimates of the liver iron stores in three large urban centres showed essentially similar results (*Charlton* et al. 1971). The condition is rare in Indians and is not found in White subjects. It first becomes manifest in late adolescence and the incidence and severity reach their greatest degree between the ages of 40 and 60 years. It appears in both sexes but males are more severely involved. *Strachan* (1929) suggested that the cause was a toxic effect of zinc and tin on the red cells. *Gillman* and *Gillman* (1945) felt that malnutrition was the basic cause resulting in the release of iron by the mitochondria. Although later *Gillman* and *Gillman* (1951) acknowledged that the excess iron was derived from the diet they claimed that it is far easier to produce an increased iron uptake and demonstrable hepatic siderosis with dietary iron overload in malnourished than in well fed animals. In 1950 *Walker* and *Arvidsson* demonstrated conclusively that the excess iron was obtained from the diet. They found the iron intake to be between 5 mg and 250 mg a day. The high content of the stools supported the dietary origin of the iron. The high content of iron in the diet is due mainly to the uptake of the element from iron utensils used during the preparation of fermented cereal products. The level of iron intake is sufficiently high to overcome the mucosal block or regulatory mechanism operating at everyday levels of intake, and allow unrequired iron to be absorbed, deposited and accumulated in the organs and tissues of the body.

Twenty four hour urine samples contain negligible quantities of iron, confirming the view that very small quantities are excreted by the kidney, even when the level of intake is several times higher than usual. Many Black subjects have a very high serum iron often associated with elevation of the total iron binding capacity with unsaturation of the iron-binding protein. It is not necessary to postulate an abnormal mechanism of iron absorption in Blacks (*Bothwell* et al. 1953) as had been suggested by *Gillman* et al. (1959). Excessive iron intake alone may be responsible for siderosis, without invoking other dietary abnormalities.

Buchanan (1972) has succeeded in producing a pathological picture of iron-overload by feeding Bantu beer to experimental animals. *Charlton* et al. (1964) suggested that alcohol itself might in addition, potentiate the absorption of iron, although it has not been possible to show an enhancement of absorption when iron has been administered in Bantu beer. It is however, possible that pancreatitis, a not infrequent occurrence in alcoholics, may be associated with excessive iron absorption due to deficiency of the exocrine secretions. This has been shown to occur in animals after pancreatectomy (*Taylor* et al. 1931), ligation of the pancreatic duct (*Taylor* et al. 1935; *Gillman* et al. 1947; *Kinney* et al. 1950), thionine induced pancreatic damage (*Kinney* et al. 1955), and in patients with chronic pancreatitis (*Davies* and *Badenach* 1962). In alcoholics with cirrhosis, iron absorption may be increased as cirrhotic subjects absorb excessive amounts of iron even when the body stores are normal or increased (*Conrad* et al. 1962). It is also possible that the suboptimal diets of many of the Blacks may potentiate iron absorption. A diet low in phosphate increases iron absorption (*Hegsted* et al. 1949).

The concentration of iron in African beer was studied by *Bothwell* et al. (1964). The average iron concentration in homebrewed African beer was 8.2 mg per 100 ml (range 0.8–15 mg per 100 ml and pH 2.23) while the average iron concentration in the beer brewed by the municipal authorities was only 1.9 mg per 100 ml (range 1.1–3.1). *Walker* and *Arvidsson* (1953) suggested that the low pH may enhance the dissolving of the iron from the container in which it is prepared. They demonstrated a high iron content in the stool of between 65 mg and 145 mg per day. The mean concentration of iron in faeces collected from males on Monday morning is several times the figure on Thursday mornings, probably reflecting weekend drinking habits. The iron absorption rate in Blacks is lower than in Whites probably because the Blacks already have varying degrees of iron overload, and an increase in the size of iron stores tends to depress absorption. However, Blacks ingesting 100 mg of iron daily absorb 2.3 mg which is quite sufficient to account for the degree of siderosis found in the middle-aged. From a quantitative point of view, the amounts absorbed daily would not have to be large to account for the deposits usually found in subjects 40 to 60 years of age. Thus daily retention in the male of 2.5 mg per day between the ages of 20 and 40 years would lead to the accumulation of 10 grams by the age of 40 which is more than the average amount in Black subjects.

Distribution of the Iron

In fully developed idiopathic haemochromatosis iron is found in large quantities in the liver and spleen and in the parenchymal cells of many of the viscera. Thus, deposits are also found in the acinar cells and islets of the pancreas, the follicular cells of the thyorid, the myofibrils of the heart, the adrenal cortex and the pituitary. *Gillman* and *Gillman* (1945) felt that the appearances in Bantu siderosis were indistinguishable from those of idiopathic haemochromatosis. *Higginson* et al. (1953) did not support this view and claimed that the iron in Bantu siderosis was confined to the liver, the spleen and reticulo-endothelial system. The higher iron content of the spleen as compared with the liver was also different from idiopathic haemochromatosis. They found an absence of pancreatic pigment in most cases, and even when haemosiderin deposits were marked in the liver and spleen, the pancreas showed only scattered iron laden macrophages in the interstitial tissue. This is in contrast to idiopathic haemochromatosis in which heavy deposits of iron in the pancreas are a feature. The absence of significant haemosiderin deposits in the epithelial elements of the stomach, thyroid, salivary and suprarenal glands and the myocardium is also in contrast to haemochromatosis. They concluded, that iron appeared in epithelial cells only when heavy deposits were present in the liver and the reticuloendothelial system. *Wainwright* (1957) supported these findings.

In a combined histopathological and chemical study, *Bothwell* and *Bradlow* (1960) confirmed the high incidence of siderosis in the adult male Black of Johannesburg and showed that siderosis first becomes manifest in late adolescence and reaches its highest degree in the forties. Eighty-nine percent of their cases showed varying degrees of hepatic siderosis. However, in 59% the siderosis was of mild degree (0.10–0.39 percent dry weight). At the other end of the scale there were 19% with iron concentrations above 1%, which is in the range found in idiopathic haemochromatosis. In their view, Bantu siderosis initially manifests in the liver parenchyma, but the splenic concentration of iron rises at the same time as the liver concentration, and with increasing levels of iron, the splenic concentration rises to higher figures than in the liver. These findings are different from those in idiopathic haemochromatosis where reticulo-endothelial deposits are not prominent, even at an advanced stage of the condition. On the other hand, this distribution is very similar to that reported in animals placed on deficient diets with heavy iron supplements. In all such studies, iron deposits have been found in the spleen and in the parenchymal and Kupffer cells of the liver relatively early in the development of iron overload. The suggested sequence is the involvement of the parenchymal cells first, followed by the Kupffer cells and finally the portal tracts (*Gillman* et al. 1959; *Bothwell* and *Bradlow* 1960), as opposed to the view that reticulo-endothelial involvement represents the earliest stage (*Higginson* et al. 1953).

Bothwell and *Isaacson* (1962) assessed the chemical iron concentrations in specimens of liver from autopsy material in 318 male and 265 female adults (Fig. 4.1).

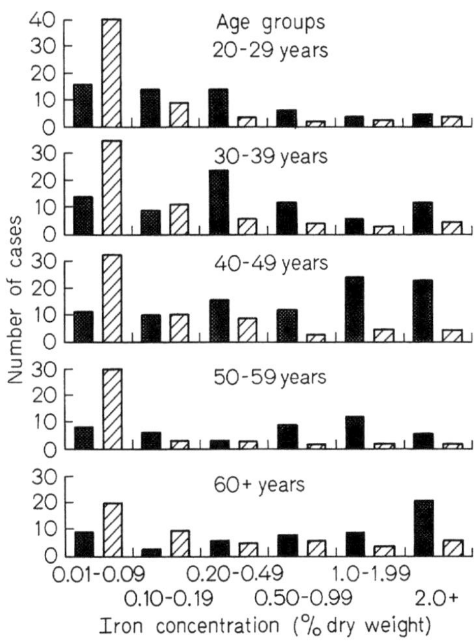

Fig. 4.1. Hepatic iron concentrations in males (black columns) and females (cross-hatched columns) at various ages. (*Bothwell* and *Isaacson* 1962)

Twenty-nine point six percent of males had liver iron concentrations which were either normal or slightly raised up to 0.19 g per 100 g dry weight. Seventy-five point four percent of females fell into this category. Thirty-seven point four percent of males and 11.6% of females had liver iron concentrations of more than 1 g per 100 g dry weight. Fifty-three subjects had between 5 and 10 g of iron in the liver and a further 35 had more than 10 g. Although there is no valid way of estimating the total body iron content in these subjects, it is probable that this would not be much higher since iron is present mainly in the liver and reticulo-endothelial system. It therefore, seems unlikely that the total body content often exceeds 15 grams. The disorder in iron balance necessary to produce this degree of iron overload is not a large one. An average absorption of 2 mg daily between the ages of 20 and 50 years would lead to a positive balance of approximately 1.4 mg daily in the male, which is quite enough to account for deposits of this magnitude. In the female, the findings are very different since about 75% had iron concentrations in the liver which were normal or very close to normal, and although severe siderosis did occur it was uncommon. A much lower incidence of iron overload in the female is probably explicable on the greater physiological losses which occur in females. It has been calculated that the average female loses up to 10 grams of iron through menstruation, pregnancy and lactation. On this basis, it must be anticipated, that the incidence and severity of iron overload would be less in females. This may not however, be the only factor. The major source of iron in the Black diet is African beer, and females, on the whole tend to drink less than males.

Large quantities are present in the spleen and when present in organs other than liver and spleen, the haemosiderin granules are to be found in macrophages and interstitial tissue only. Iron is not usually present in the parenchymal cells of organs other than the liver. Thus in the pancreas, adrenal, pituitary, thyroid and heart, small quantities may be found in the interstitial tissue or in macrophages. Iron in the reticulo-endothelial cells of the marrow may be a prominent feature. Even in the presence of severe overload, iron is usually confined to the liver and reticulo-endothelial system. This pattern is therefore, different from idiopathic haemochromatosis, but is very similar to what is found in animals placed on deficient diets with heavy iron supplements. There is however, a percentage of cases in which iron pigment appears in the parenchymal cells of organs other than the liver including the acinar and islets cells of the pancreas, the follicular cells of the thyroid and the myofibrils of the heart. These cases usually have an associated cirrhosis (*Isaacson* et al. 1961) although an occasional instance has been observed in which the liver shows marked portal tract fibrosis without fully developed cirrhosis. Examples of the latter are however, rare and in most cases of significant parenchymal iron in viscera other than the liver, cirrhosis is present. *Isaacson* et al. (1961) showed that subjects with severe siderosis but without cirrhosis had remarkably high concentrations of iron in the liver and spleen, the average in the liver being 2.21% dry weight and in the spleen 3.38%.

The concentration in the other organs was however negligible and iron was confined to the reticulo-endothelial cells and never found in the parenchymal cells. The subjects in this group died of a variety of diseases quite unrelated to the degree of iron overload, although it may be of some significance that a large percentage died of tuberculosis. *Buchanan* (1970) has suggested that the virulence of organisms may be enhanced by iron. In subjects with macronodular cirrhosis the average levels of iron in liver and spleen were similar to apparent normals in the same age groups.

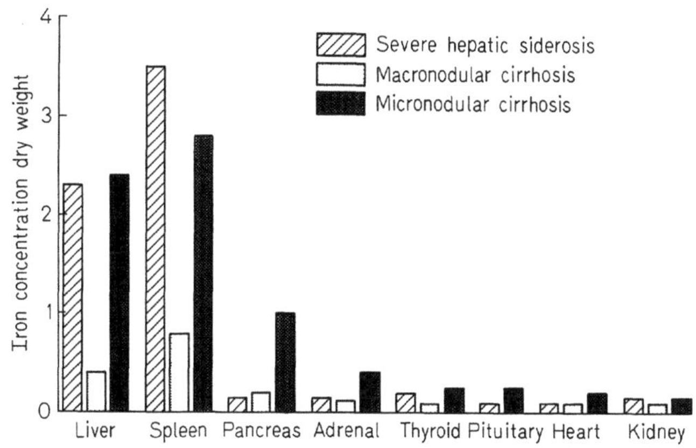

Fig. 4.2

In only one case were iron deposits present in parenchymal cells other than the liver. Striking findings were present in the group with micronodular cirrhosis. Excessive deposits of iron in the liver were found in all except two cases, one of which was grossly fatty, and the livers were macroscopically brown due to the iron. The average iron concentration in the liver was 2.31% and spleen 2.63%. There were heavy iron deposits in the pancreas, heart, thyroid, adrenal and pituitary, and histologically, excessive quantitites of iron were found not only in the liver and spleen but also in the parenchymal cells of the pancreas in which the acini and islets were deeply pigmented, the follicular cells of the thyroid, the myofibrils of the heart, the adrenal glands (where the zona glomerulosa showed the severest involvement) and the pituitary.

The histological findings in this group were therefore, véry similar to those of idiopathic haemochromatosis. Figure 4.2 summarizes the biochemical findings in these three groups (*Isaacson* et al. 1961). Excessive deposits of iron play no part in the pathogenesis of macronodular cirrhosis and when they occur simultaneously, it is only because varying degrees of iron overload are so common in Blacks. Iron overloaded beer is not an aetiological factor in macronodular cirrhosis.

Cases of micronodular cirrhosis show severe iron overload of the liver, the reticulo-endothelial system and other parenchymal tissues, the only feature serving to distinguish these cases from idiopathic haemochromatosis being the relatively high splenic concentration. In micronodular cirrhosis parenchymal iron is present in other organs irrespective of the amount of iron in the liver or spleen, some livers with micronodular cirrhosis and heavy pancreatic deposits having less iron than those cases with severe siderosis and no cirrhosis in which pancreatic deposits are absent. In occasional instances the iron concentration in the pancreas is higher than in the liver. Widespread parenchymal deposits of iron are therefore, a consequence of the development of cirrhosis (*Isaacson* et al. 1961; *Bradlow* et al. 1961) and are not an "overflow" phenomenon from an already overloaded reticulo-endothelial system (*Higginson* et al. 1953; *Wainwright* 1957). The distribution of iron overload in other parenchymal tissues takes place in a regular sequence, the heaviest deposits being found in the pancreas, followed by the adrenals, thyroid, pituitary and heart. The pattern of widespread parenchymal deposits does not seem to be related to the type of cirrhosis as it was also found in one case of macronodular cirrhosis with severe hepatic siderosis. The explanation of these findings is obscure. Internal Eck fistulae in the cirrhotic liver might shunt much of the iron-containing portal blood past the liver directly into the general circulation. Transferrin levels tend to be lower when cirrhosis is present but percentage saturation is high. There is experimental evidence that iron is taken up more readily by parenchymal tissues under such circumstances (*Schwartz* 1956). *Buchanan* (1969) exposed human tissue in the test tube to transferrin saturated 50% and 90% respectively with radio active iron, and in all instances the tissues of epithelial origin took up the transferrin in a significantly greater amount from the 90% saturated sample. In Blacks with siderosis and cirrhosis, the percentage saturation of the circulating transferrin is raised, whereas with siderosis but no cirrhosis the percentage saturation is normal.

Folic acid deficiency may also play a part in the distribution of iron, in that experimentally an iron rich diet associated with folic acid deficiency produces extrahepatic parenchymal iron deposits (*MacDonald* et al. 1965). Whatever the explanation for these findings, there is no doubt that a proportion of Black adults with cirrhosis develops a pathological picture virtually indistinguishable from idiopathic haemochromatosis. Rarely this may occur in the absence of cirrhosis, but in these cases the degree of fibrosis is such as to probably compromise the metabolic functions of the liver. A further point in relation to the distribution of iron concerns its site of deposition in the liver. *Higginson* et al. (1953) claimed that the initial deposit is always in the Kupffer cells, and that only subsequently does iron appear in the hepatic cells. Other authors (*Gillman* and *Gillman* 1951; *Wainwright* 1957; *Bothwell* and *Bradlow* 1960) did not support this view. In most cases with iron concentrations between 0.1% and 0.4%, haemosiderin granules are present in parenchymal cells. Between 0.4% and 0.6%, moderate amounts are present in parenchymal cells and minimal deposits in Kupffer cells and, with increasing concentrations, increasing amounts appear in liver cells, Kupffer cells and portal tracts (*Bothwell* and *Bradlow* 1960).

Effect of the Iron

Considerable controversy exists as to whether the iron is harmful or not, some workers claiming no pathological effects of iron overload (*Rather* 1956). In idiopathic haemochromatosis there is dispute about the role iron plays in the production of tissue damage, and many authorities claim that the pathological changes found could equally well be a direct result of the metabolic defect that leads to excessive iron absorption rather than to the irritative effect of iron itself. The pathological effects of iron overload will be considered under the following headings: (1) Liver, (2) Pancreas, (3) Bones, (4) Miscellaneous.

Effect on the Liver

The early workers thought that cirrhosis and siderosis were not causally related (*Gillman* et al. 1945; *Higginson* et al. 1953; *Wainwright* 1957). However, later studies (*Higginson* et al. 1957; *Gillman* et al. 1958; *Bothwell* and *Bradlow* 1960) showed a close correlation between portal fibrosis and cirrhosis with advanced siderosis.

Bothwell and *Isaacson* (1962) found portal fibrosis or cirrhosis very common in both male and female subjects with liver iron concentrations of more than 2 g per 100 g. They suggested that as fibrosis is not present in all such cases there were other factors which could potentiate the fibrogenic effects of excessive iron deposits. Apart from the toxic effects of the alcohol itself, these beverages contain numerous unidentified adulterants. It has also been shown experimentally that the liver overloaded with iron is very vulnerable to toxic, nutritional and metabolic hazards, and such factors may aggravate the effects of the iron deposits (*Golberg* and *Smith* 1960).

A significant correlation between siderosis and micronodular cirrhosis was demonstrated by several authors (*Gillman* et al. 1957; *Isaacson* et al. 1961). In a series of 24 micronodular cirrhoses, *Isaacson* et al. (1961) demonstrated severe hepatic deposits of iron in all except two cases. The average hepatic iron concentration in this group was 2.31% (range 0.07–8.16). The mean concentration was approximately twice as great as occurs at comparable ages in the general population. No association was however, found between iron overload and macronodular cirrhosis.

Effect on the Pancreas

Originally it was thought that the association of diabetes mellitus and siderosis occurred extremely rarely in Blacks (*Higginson* et al. 1953; *Wainwright* 1957). It was the observation by *Isaacson* et al. (1961) that cases of micronodular cirrhosis and siderosis often showed heavy parenchymal iron deposits in the pancreas, that stimulated a closer study of the autopsy records of Black diabetics. Twenty cases were studied and in 7 no demonstrable iron in any organ was found, while in 6 there was mild liver siderosis but no deposits in other epithelial tissues (*Seftel* et al. 1960).

One subject showed heavy liver siderosis but no cirrhosis, and iron was not present in other parenchymal tissues. In 2 further cases tissues were not available for analysis but the full autopsy records available made it clear that siderosis was not a feature in either. In the remaining four subjects there was micronodular cirrhosis with siderosis and widespread parenchymal iron deposits in the pancreas, thyroid, heart, adrenal and pituitary. These observations were confirmed by chemical analyses. Thus in four of the twenty cases the histological and chemical findings resembled those seen in idiopathic haemochromatosis. Although it was theoretically possible that these subjects were suffering from the genetic disorder, there were several reasons which made such a possibility untenable. In the first place, the number found in this series would suggest an incidence of the disease far in excess of that described elsewhere. Secondly, the concentrations of iron in the spleen were generally greater than those described in the genetic disorder. These were clearly cases of severe siderosis with cirrhosis and secondary pancreatic involvement – examples of diabetes induced by the ingestion of excessive quantities of iron. A subsequent in vivo study of 100 Black diabetics was undertaken to assess what proportion was suffering from diabetes due to iron overload (*Seftel* et al. 1961). Plasma iron levels were estimated in all subjects. Ten men and 4 women had levels above 150 micrograms per 100 ml. Liver biopsies were carried out on eleven of these subjects. In four men and three women the liver biopsies showed marked siderosis with micronodular cirrhosis. In view of the known association of iron deposits in the pancreas with siderosis and cirrhosis of the liver, these 7 cases were regarded as being examples of diabetes due to severe siderosis with cirrhosis and secondary pancreatic involvement. This was confirmed histologically and chemically in two who subsequently died. A comparison of a group of these diabetics with a random group of 100 diabetics with normal plasma iron levels, showed several differences. The iron overloaded group was generally underweight and wasted. They all showed signs of severe liver disease and always gave a history of having consumed large quantities of home brewed alcohol. Hepatomegaly, with features of portal hypertension and liver failure were present. Common complications were tuberculosis and porphyria cutanea tarda with increased urinary excretion of uroporphyrins. The diabetes was difficult to control, often severe, with hypoglycaemic attacks. The severe associated liver disease gives the diabetics a very poor prognosis. The control group was generally obese, did not show signs of liver disease and gave an alcoholic history in only one fifth of the cases. Most of the iron overloaded group were males, whereas the control group showed a female to male ratio of 1.8:1. The combination of liver disease and the severity of the diabetes contributes to a much poorer prognosis in the group with iron overload and cirrhosis. Based on this investigation it appears that approximately 7% of Black diabetics are subjects with siderosis and cirrhosis. This incidence is extremely high when compared with the 0.16% incidence of idiopathic haemochromatosis in an American series of thirty thousand diabetic subjects. As compared with the idiopathic disease, the Black diabetics with iron overload and cirrhosis show a much more rapid downhill course, liver failure dominating the clinical picture. Cardiac complications are not a feature. This is not surprising as it had been shown that the heart is one of the last organs to accumulate iron deposits in African siderosis, cirrhosis generally causing death before they have reached significant proportions.

Effect on the Bones

For many years it had been recognized that collapse of lumber vertebrae occurs commonly in middle aged Blacks (*Walker* et al. 1955; *Grusin* and *Samuel* 1957), that the collapse was due to osteoporosis and that these patients are all severely siderotic (*Seftel* et al. 1963). *Seftel* et al. (1966) then described the association of osteoporosis, scurvy and siderosis. Fourteen of their patients showed signs of scurvy and all consumed large quantities of African beer. They suggested that the siderosis might give rise to scurvy by the rapid oxidative catabolism of any absorbed ascorbic acid (*Mazur* and *Sackler* 1967).

Bothwell et al. (1964) showed that scorbutic adults usually have severe siderosis and that it is very difficult to saturate such subjects with ascorbic acid. It had been suggested that when siderotic individuals subsist on a borderline diet, the available ascorbic acid is irreversibly oxidized by the large deposits of ferric iron (*Lynch* et al. 1967). It is known that ascorbic acid is necessary for the formation of bone matrix, and that guinea pigs maintained on a diet low in ascorbic acid develop osteoporosis (*Hojer* 1923). A proportion of malnourished siderotic Blacks therefore develops osteoporosis as a result of irreversible oxidation of available ascorbic acid by the iron deposits (*Seftel* et al. 1964). Clinically, the main symptom is low back pain, but vertebral or even femoral head collapse may result. Most of these patients are manual labourers, almost all drink large quantities of their traditional alcoholic beverages, they are almost invariably severely siderotic, and they usually show clinical or biochemical evidence of vitamin C deficiency (*Lynch* et al. 1967). *Lynch* et al. (1967) investigated 110 asymptomatic manual labourers whose diet contained large amounts of iron and little ascorbic acid. The mean leucocyte ascorbic acid concentration of this group was significantly lower than that of the control group and fifteen percent of these subjects showed radiological evidence of vertebral osteoporosis. In a further group of 71 Black males dying of acute trauma, there was a significant inverse correlation between the mineral density of the iliac crest bone and the hepatic iron concentration. Osteoporosis occurs both in scorbutic children and experimentally in animals. *Wapnick* et al. (1971) demonstrated that in vitamin C deficient guinea pigs, there is not only a decrease in bone formation, but also an increase in bone resorption, and this has also been demonstrated in osteoporotic Blacks with severe iron overload.

Ascorbic acid deficiency is rare in Negro infants, whereas biochemical evidence of ascorbic acid deficiency in clinical scurvy is common in adults with siderosis (*Seftel* et al. 1966). Repeated administration of large doses of ascrobic acid to normal subjects results in most of the vitamin being excreted in the urine unchanged, whereas in iron overloaded individuals the vitamin C is oxidized to oxalic acid by the ferric iron in the tissues and the urinary excretion of oxalic acid increases markedly (*Lynch* et al. 1967; *Schultz* and *Swanepoel* 1962). White subjects with iron overload of diverse aetiology also show low leucocyte ascorbic acid levels (*Wapnick* et al. 1968, 1970, 1971). *Wapnick* et al. (1970) have pointed out that serum iron can be used as an index of iron overload in Blacks only after repletion with ascorbic acid. Therapy, with ascorbic acid raises the mean serum iron level in a siderotic group. When this is done, there is a highly significant correlation between the levels of serum iron and the marrow iron grading. The association of spinal osteoporosis, siderosis and scurvy as seen in South Africa has not been reported from Zimbabwe but appears to occur in Zambia.

The observation associating iron overload with vertebral deformities is not new, as a syndrome with similar features was described almost a century ago in Manchuria in people who derive the excess iron from well water. In New Zealand, cattle which are siderotic, develop severe osteoporosis (*Hartley* 1959), and in this area the drinking water has a high iron content. Guinea pigs overloaded with iron by injections of iron dextran develop significantly reduced hepatic ascorbic acid concentrations and bone mineral densities. The percentage bone formation surface is significantly diminished and the percentage bone resorption surface significantly increased. Ascorbic acid injections largely prevent the bone changes (*Wapnick* et al. 1971).

Miscellaneous

Porphyria Cutanea Tarda

Keeley (1964) reported that over a 15 year period at Baragwanath Hospital he had seen only one case of congenital erythropoietic porphyria, but patients with acquired porphyria (porphyria cutanea tarda) accounted for five of every one thousand medical admissions. No case of acute intermittent porphyria, variegate porphyria or protoporphyria erythropoietica had yet been encountered in a Black. The frequency of acquired porphyria in Black patients was also emphasized by an outpatient survey which showed an incidence of 13 cases per thousand adult outpatients. The ratio of males to females was 1.3:1, and all cases encountered were over 25 years of age. Clinically, these patients presented with hyper pigmentation, scars on the hands, facial hirsutes and occasionally active bullae. In 25 patients admitted to the wards with acquired porphyria, striking findings were hepatomegaly with siderosis, heavy alcohol consumption, cirrhosis in a high percentage and diabetes in two out of twenty five cases. Of nine diabetics with cirrhosis and iron overload three had porphyria. When 100 control diabetics with a normal serum iron concentration were screened, only two were found to have porphyria, suggesting that porphyria is commoner when the diabetes is associated with iron overload. African siderosis is now a recognized association of acquired cutaneous porphyria, and an important factor is the habitual ingestion of alcohol drinks of high iron content to which adulterants are often added (*Seftel* 1964).

Disturbances in iron metabolism have been noted in several types of porphyria. Excessive accumulation of iron in the reticulo-endothelial system has been found in erythropoietic porphyria, and also in symptomatic porphyria, as seen both in Black and White subjects. In addition, high plasma iron levels have been reported in the acute phase of porphyria variegata.

Although the association between siderosis in Blacks and symptomatic porphyria seems a definite one, its significance is less certain. The subjects who develop iron overload derive most of this iron from the containers used in the preparation of home-brewed alcoholic drinks, so that the gross degrees of tissue siderosis tend to occur in those subjects drinking the most alcohol. It is therefore feasible, that the siderosis is not casually related to symptomatic porphyria, but that both are the end results of the peculiar drinking habits. The association between iron overload and symptomatic porphyria has not only been noted in Blacks, but has been reported in White subjects, generally males who consume a great deal of alcohol and in whom diabetes in not an uncommon complication. The fact that patients with symptomatic porphyria exhibit clinical and pathological features similar to those described in Blacks suggests that the conditions have a common aetiological basis. The White subjects may accumulate iron in the body as a result of several mechanisms. The iron intake in alcoholics may be quite high since iron is found in a significant amount in many wines (*MacDonald* 1963). In addition a high proportion of alcoholic subjects have chronic liver disease and chronic pancreatitis, both of which increase iron absorption from the bowel. In addition, alcohol itself may increase iron absorption (*Charlton* et al. 1964).

Whether the presence of excessive iron deposits has any influence on the subsequent development of symptomatic porphyria in Black and White subjects has not been settled. Generally symptomatic porphyria is not a feature of either classical idiopathic haemochromatosis or transfusional siderosis. *Lamont* and *Hathorn* (1960) found increased plasma iron in Blacks with porphyria. In addition, they found liver changes in many of their Black porphyrics varying from minor alterations in the intralobular and periportal reticulum framework, to gross distortion of lobular architecture with scarring, hyperplastic nodules and cirrhosis. *Lamont* et al. (1961) showed that in most cases fibrotic lesions of the liver are present and that most of the liver contains iron.

Since *Barnes* (1945) first described a series of cases in South African Blacks, the number of cases of porphyria has multiplied rapidly (*Kramer* 1963). There is no basic difference in the clinical pattern in porphyria in Blacks from that seen in Whites, but acute intermittent cases are very rare, the vast majority being benign and showing the characteristic skin lesions of chronic cutaneous porphyria (*Shaper* 1958). Approximately one third present with characteristic blistering skin lesions, but the remainder present for reasons bearing no relation to porphyria. Generally darkening of the skin over the face and hands is common and in some cases the diagnosis of pellagra may be made. The Africans in Zimbabwe regard the condition as being due to drinking excessive quantities of beer (*Gelfand* 1955). The liver in acquired porphyria, may show siderosis, focal necrosis, portal fibrosis and cirrhosis (*Uys* and *Eales* 1963). The association of cirrhotic liver disease accompanied by moderate siderosis and acquired porphyria is a real one (*Bolgert* et al. 1953; *Galambos* 1975). *Keeley* et al. (1960) reported on liver biopsies carried out on 25 Black subjects with symptomatic porphyria cutanea tarda. In 22 there were varying degrees of siderosis and in 8 cirrhosis was present. Rats previously rendered siderotic by intraperitoneal administration of iron dextran, become porphyric much more rapidly than non siderotic animals when fed hexachlorobenzene (*Taljaard* et al. 1972), and there is an increasing liver iron in rats rendered porphyric by hexochlorobenzene (*Campbell* 1963). Ethanol has been shown to be capable of increasing porphyrin synthesis and excretion in this disease, thus suggesting that its role is that of an aggravating factor. On the other hand, the part played by hepatic iron overload is not at all clear. Iron accelerates the porphyrinogenic activity of hexachlorobenzene, and high serum iron values with marked transferrin saturation have been reported in porphyria cutanea tarda (*Epstein* and *Pinsky* 1965).

Porphyrin synthesis in human porcine crude liver extracts is greatly stimulated by ferrous iron and the porphyrin produced is chiefly uroporphyrinogen 1 (*Kushner* et al. 1971). The action of ferrous iron is that of a direct inhibitory effect on the enzyme Cosyn (cosynthetase). Thus ferrous iron produces a biochemical change in liver extract that appears identical to the in vivo defect of porphyria cutanea tarda. Iron overload has been implicated in the pathogenesis of porphyria cutanea tarda on the basis of three observations. First, hepatic cell iron loading is almost invariably found in patients with the disorder; second, removal of iron by phlebotomy or the administration of iron chelating agents induces both clinical and biochemical remissions in such patients (*Epstein* and *Redeker* 1968). Finally, the administration of iron is followed by relapse in patients in whom remission had been induced by phlebotomy therapy (*Felsher* and *Redeker* 1972). The effects of iron are due to its inhibitory action on Cosyn. It is however, important to realise that iron overload alone does not induce porphyria cutanea tarda, nor does iron content alone induce abnormal porphyrin synthesis. Conversion to the ferrous form is required. Thus the in vivo development of porphyria cutanea tarda may depend partly on iron overload and partly on the presence of a system capable of reducing iron.

Infection Shock and Iron Overload

Buchanan (1970) reported 21 cases of peritonitis in Black subjects at autopsy and in none of these was there a primary focus of infection, and all but one had marked siderosis. He suggested that there was a casual relationship between advanced degrees of siderosis and unexplained peritonitis and that grossly excessive iron stores lower the body's resistance to infection as result of blocking of the reticulo-endothelial system by large inert iron containing molecules. *Gillman* and *Gillman* (1951) originally suggested that the rapid progress of tuberculosis in Blacks may similarly be due to blocking of the reticulo-endothelial system by particles. Similar types of peritonitis have been described in haemochromatosis (*Jones* 1962). In a later publication *Buchanan* (1971) reported five patients with iron overload who died in severe shock for which there was no obvious cause. He suggested that the shock was septic in nature as a result of enhancement of the virulence of enteric organisms by iron present in large amounts in patients with African siderosis or idiopathic haemochromatosis. *Jones* (1962) described irreversible shock in hameochromatosis, and shock is a fairly well recognized complication of this disease. In the cases described by *Buchanan* (1971), all but one had a very high serum iron and acute liver cell necrosis. The degree of shock and liver cell necrosis correlated well with the height of the serum iron. *Buchanan* feels that the mechanism of shock may not be the conventionally accepted one of massive release of ferritin into the circulation from necrotic liver cells causing vasodilatation, but that the shock in patients with excessive iron stores is a septic shock due to gram negative bacteraemia. This septic shock is frequently associated with infection of the peritoneal cavity and in some instances the underlying pathology is that of a phlegmonous colitis producing a markedly oedematous colon. Iron compounds can enhance the virulence of some organisms (*Murray* et al. 1980) and *Buchanan* suggested that in certain circumstances gram negative bacteria from the bowel, whose virulence has been enhanced by the iron, may invade the body to produce peritonitis and septic shock. Iron lessens the efficacy of some anti-tuberculosis drugs (*Martin* et al. 1963) and *Buchanan* (1972) also suggests that the prevalence of tuberculosis in advanced siderotics is high, and that the iron may make anti-tuberculous drugs less effective.

Tightness of the Skin over the Feet and Lower Limbs

Forbes (1966) reported three cases of Bantu siderosis presenting with painful lower limbs in which there was tightness of the skin over the feet and lower limbs. He suggested a relationship between these two conditions and that patients presenting with pain and skin tightness should be investigated for iron overload. The mechanism is obscure.

Pathological Findings in Iron Overload

Excellent descriptions of the pathology of siderosis in Blacks are to be found in the literature (*Higginson* et al. 1953; *Wainwright* 1957), and the findings will be freely quoted.

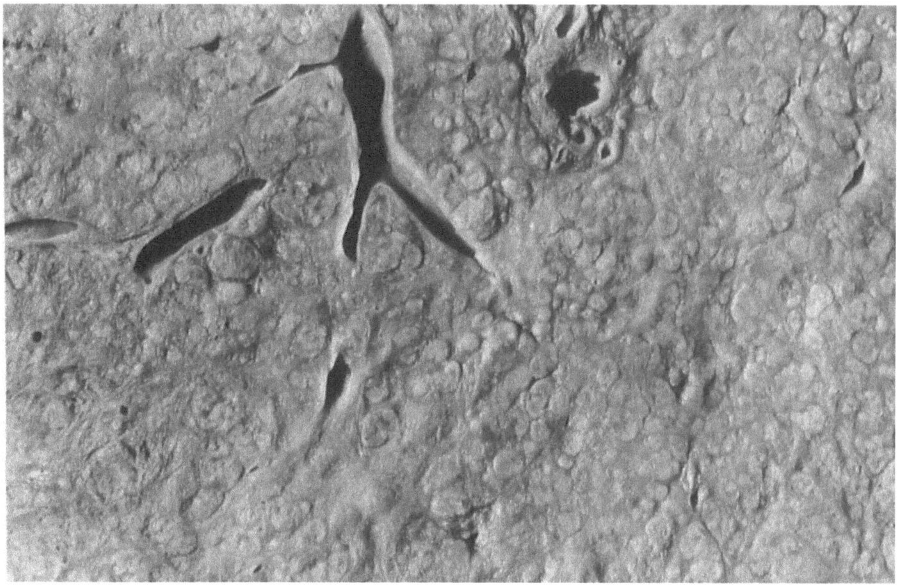

Fig. 4.3. Typical micronodular cirrhosis with iron overload. The nodules are small and do not generally exceed 3 mm in diameter

The description which follows applies to the majority of subjects with iron overload, and particularly to those without cirrhosis. With the development of cirrhosis there may be an alteration in the distribution of iron and a change in the pathological picture.

Externally, no significant abnormalities can be found in most subjects with iron overload. In a few instances, microscopic examination of the skin may show a few scattered haemosiderin granules, but this is not a constant feature, and it bears no relationship to the amount of iron in the liver or spleen.

The Liver

This organ generally has a rusty brown colour but the weight does not appear to be affected by the amount of iron present. Generally when cirrhosis is present with severe iron overload, the cirrhosis is of the micronodular type (Fig. 4.3). In occasional cases, a macronodular cirrhosis is present, but in such circumstances the presence of iron overload appears to be coincidental. Microscopically, in the early stages, the iron is present in the periportal zone of the lobule at the biliary pole of the liver cells (*Wainwright* 1957).

The pigmentation progressively advances to the centre of the lobule until all the parenchymal cells contain iron pigment, and in the next stage clumps of pigment appear in the portal tracts. The earliest involvement is of the parenchymal cells, followed by the Kupffer cells and finally the portal tracts. When Kupffer cells are heavily

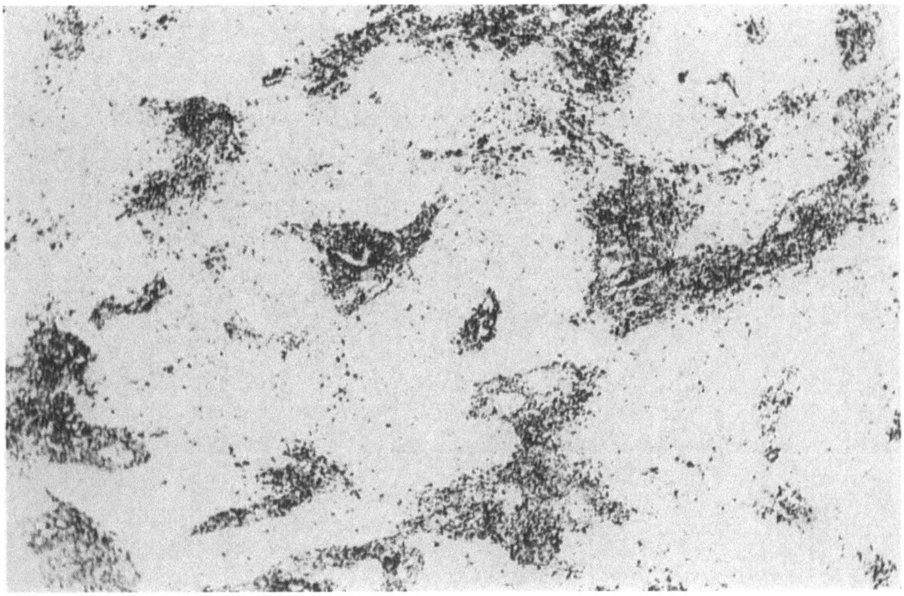

Fig. 4.4. Low power view of ironoverloaded liver with increased portal tract fibrosis but no cirrhosis. Perl's Prussian blue, × 24

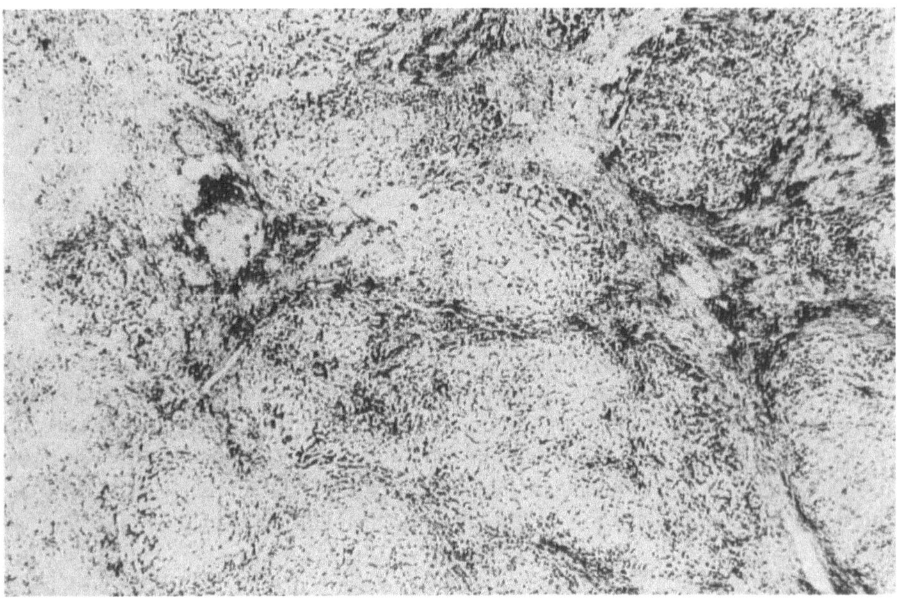

Fig. 4.5. Section of liver with micronodular cirrhosis and marked iron overload. Perl's Prussian blue, × 90

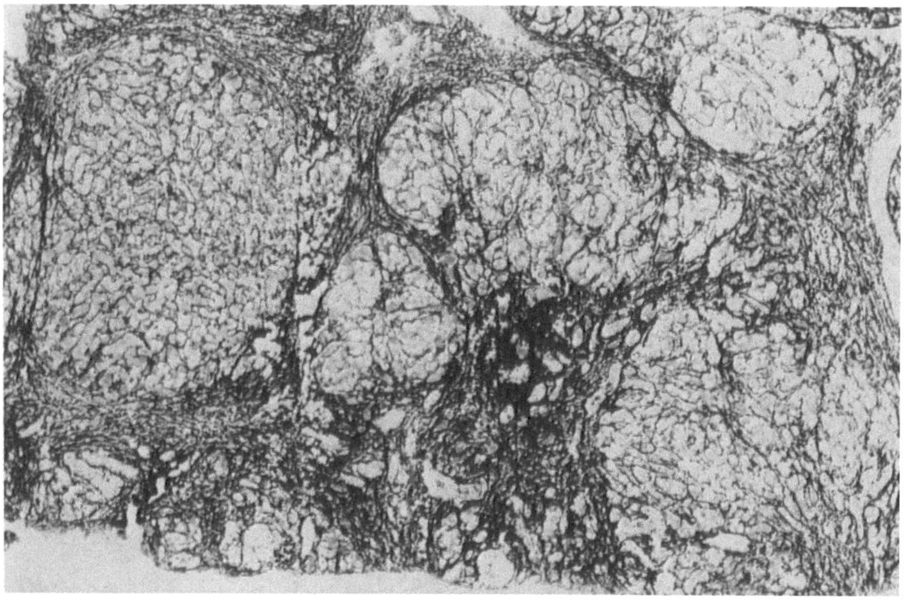

Fig. 4.6. Reticulin impregnation demonstrating micronodular cirrhosis. Sweet's reticulin, ×70

loaded with iron, large granules of pigment obscure the nuclear detail. The heavy deposits of iron do not appear to damage the liver cells. Occasional groups of hepatocytes devoid of haemosiderin can be seen. This indicates regeneration and a similar appearance is observed in the centres of regenerating nodules in cirrhosis. With increasing degrees of iron overload, very heavy deposits are present in the portal tracts. These vary from ironladen macrophages to heavy intracellular and extracellular masses. Not infrequently, the epithelium of the small bile ducts contains large amount of haemosiderin, and in addition iron granules can be seen in the endothelial cells of the portal blood vessels (Figs. 4.4–4.7). Some of the liver cells also contain a second brownish non iron containing pigment known as lipochrome (*Wainwright* 1957).

The Spleen

The iron concentration of the spleen rises paripassu with that of the liver, and with marked iron overload, the concentration of iron in the spleen exceeds that of the liver. Macroscopically, the spleen in siderotic cases shows a rusty colour. In some instances of mild iron overload the liver may appear macroscopically normal but the spleen shows a distinct brownish discolouration. In the milder cases of iron overload, iron is present in the endothelial cells and macrophages and with increasing concentrations of iron, the number of iron-laden macrophages in the pulp rises, to form dense masses some of which appear extracellular (Fig. 4.8).

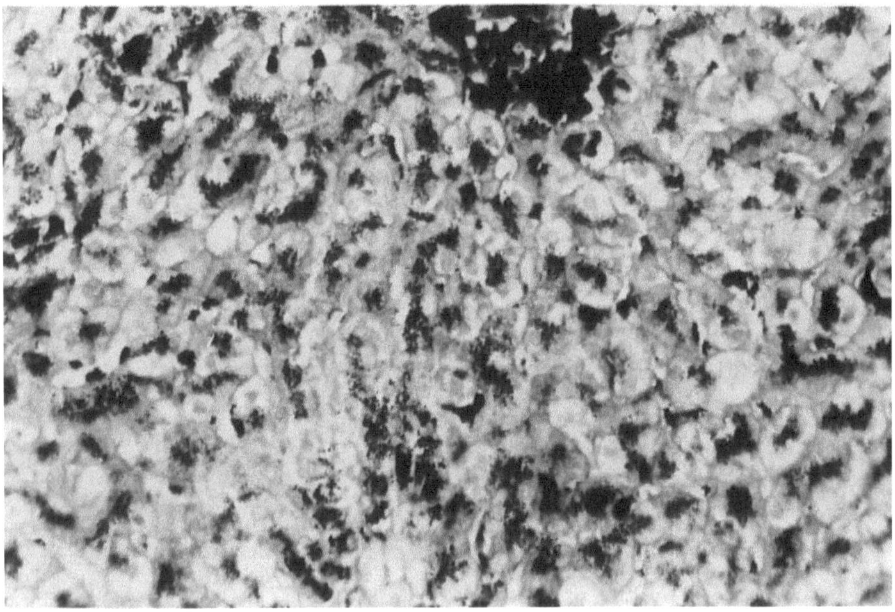

Fig. 4.7. High power view of liver with marked iron overload. Perl's Prussian blue, ×285

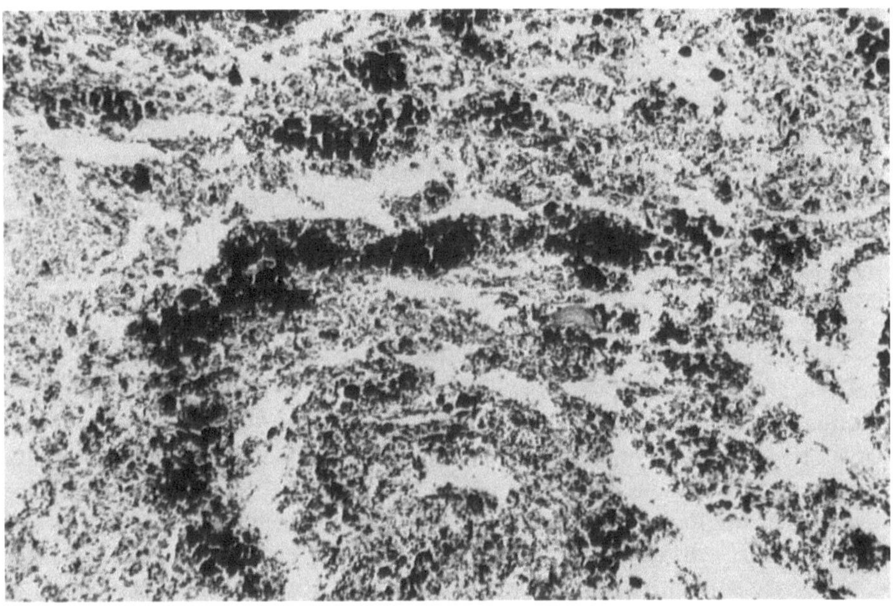

Fig. 4.8. Spleen showing heavy iron overload. Perl's Prussian blue, ×95

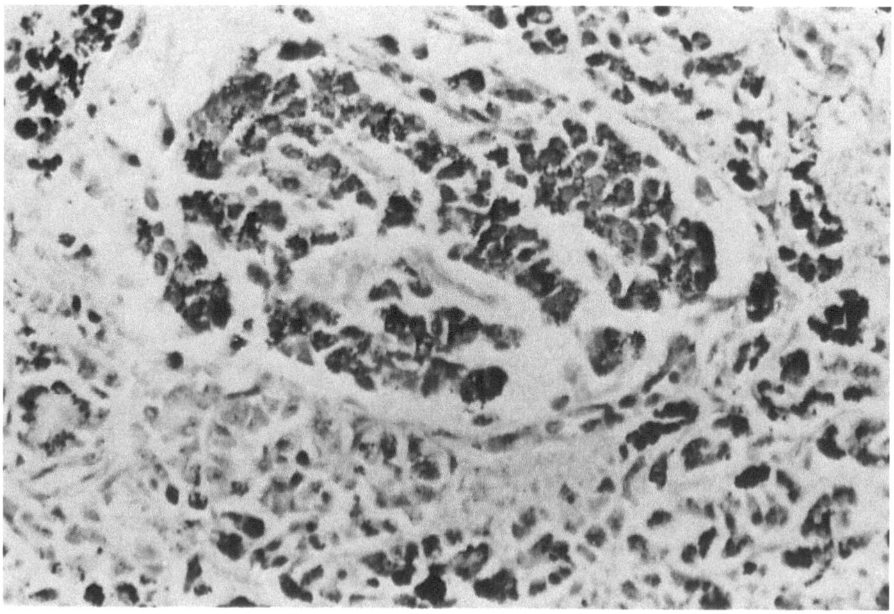

Fig. 4.9. Pancreas in case of cirrhosis with marked iron overload. Haemosiderin granules are present in acinar cells and islets. Perl's Prussian blue, ×420

Iron-laden histiocytes can also be found in the capsule and trabeculae, and the endothelium of the trabecular veins frequently contains haemosiderin granules. Generally, the iron deposits are less prominent in the malpighian corpuscles.

Pancreas

Macroscopically, the pancreas usually appears normal. In subjects with cirrhosis in which the distribution of iron is altered, the pancreas may present a brownish colour. In cases with iron overload and no cirrhosis, the pancreas may show small quantities of iron, but this is confined to the reticulo-endothelial system, with iron laden macrophages in the interstitial tissue. Parenchymal iron deposits in the pancreas occur in the presence of cirrhosis, but there are occasional instances in which iron deposits are present in the parenchymal cells in the absence ofovert cirrhosis. When parenchymal deposits of iron are present they are seen in both the acinar cells and the islets of Langerhans (Fig. 4.9).

The Heart

The heart generally shows no significant changes. In occasional cases there may be a few granules of haemosiderin in the interstitial tissue, but only rarely are granules

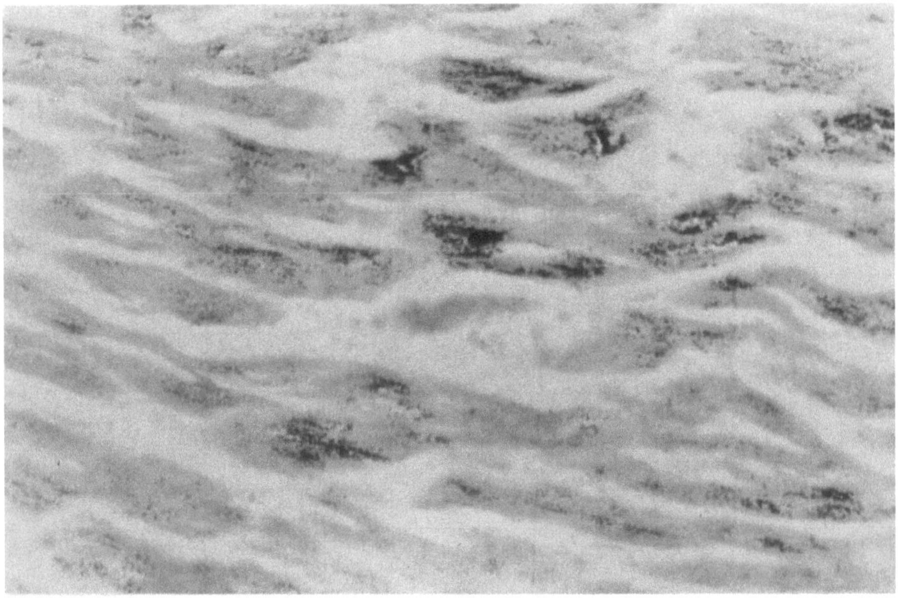

Fig. 4.10. Myofibrils containing haemosiderin granules in case of iron overload with cirrhosis. Perl's Prussian blue, ×415

found in the myofibrils themselves. In some instances of cirrhosis with iron overload however, haemosiderin may be found within the myofibrils (Fig. 4.10).

The Kidney

Scanty haemosiderin granules are often found in the distal convoluted tubules and also in the loops of Henle. In some cases, small granules of iron pigment are also present in the glomerular tufts. Iron-laden macrophages are present in the interstitial tissue.

The Gastro Intestinal Tract

The most striking feature on opening the bowel is the deep rusty brown colour of the duodenal and jejunal mucosa due to heavy pigmentation of the substantia propria of the villi. The lymph nodes draining these portions of the bowel are pigmented. The stomach, ileum and colon are usually normal. The rusty brown colour of the bowel in iron overload is most intense in the third and fourth parts of the duodenum and upper jejunum, and then diminishes and disappears in the lower jejunum and ileum. Microscopic examination shows iron laden macrophages in the substantia propria of the villi, and in severe cases all cellular detail in the villi is obscured by masses of intracellular and extracellular pigment (Fig. 4.11). Similar changes are present in the duodenum, but Brunner's glands are not usually involved (*Higginson* et al. 1953). A rise in the con-

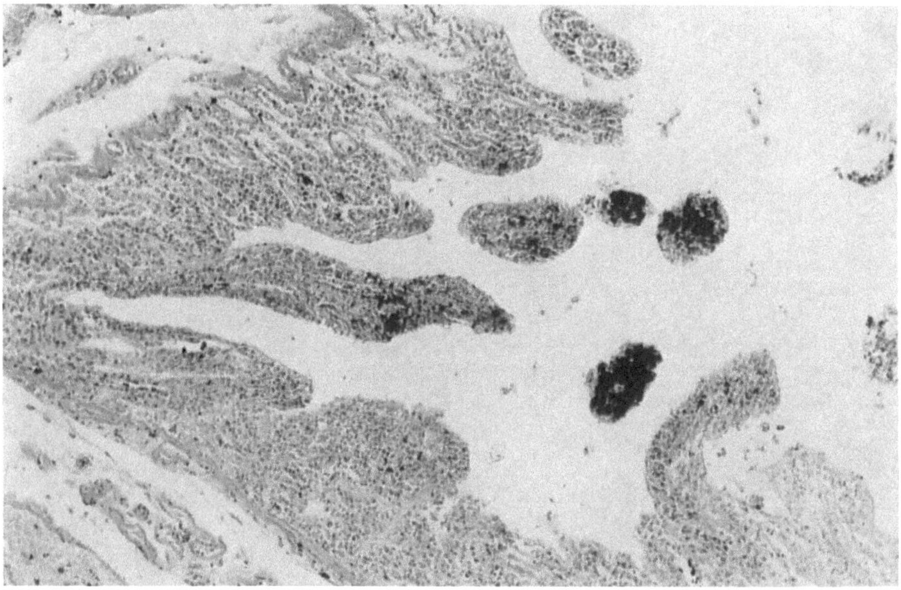

Fig. 4.11. Low power view of haemosiderin granules in the duodenal villi. Perl's Prussian blue, ×90

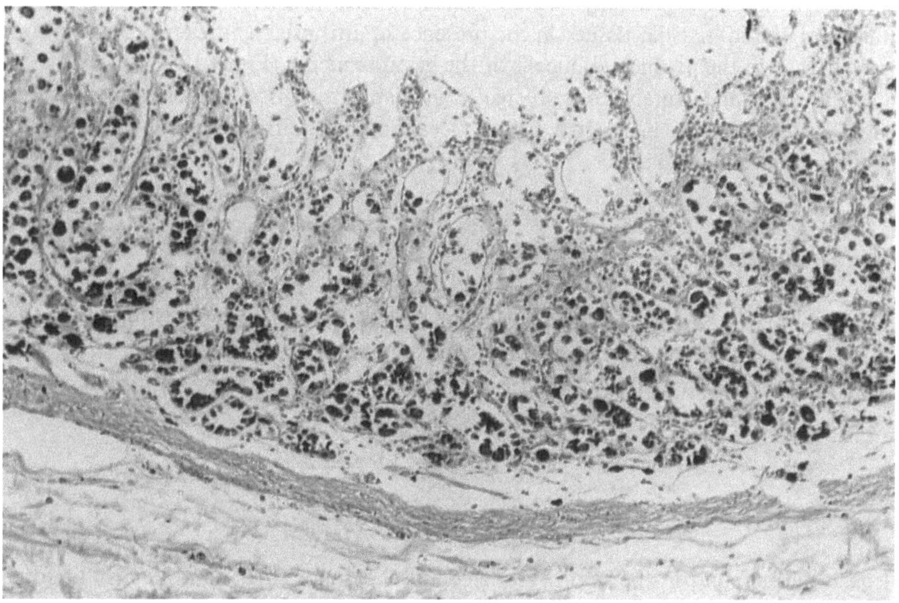

Fig. 4.12. Section of stomach in subject with marked iron overload and cirrhosis. Perl's Prussian blue, ×90

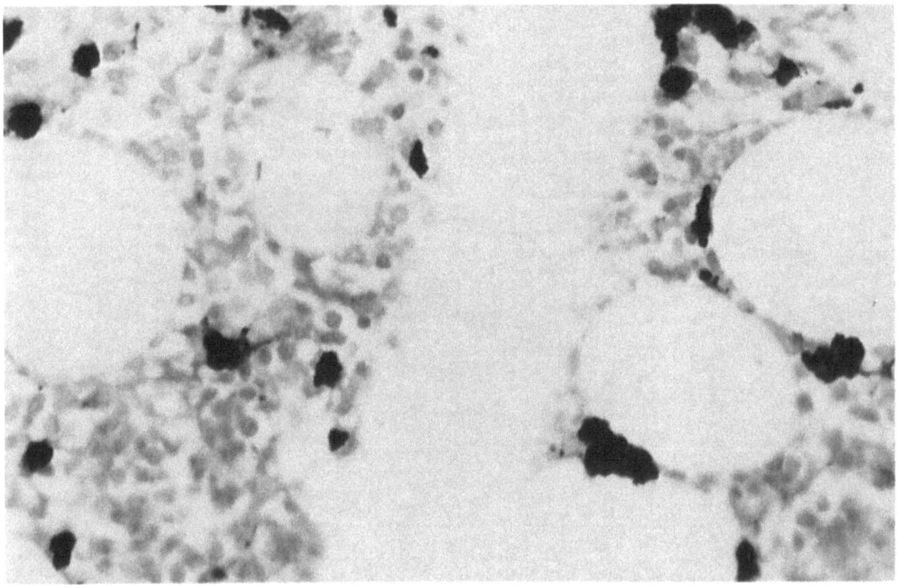

Fig. 4.13. Haemosiderin granules in bone marrow. Perl's Prussian blue, ×415

centration of iron in the jejunum usually accompanies an increase in the liver and spleen. The stomach generally contains small quantities of haemosiderin in the macrophages of the interstitial tissue. In the presence of cirrhosis significant deposits of iron may be seen in the parenchymal cells of the gastric mucosa (Fig. 4.12).

Salivary glands rarely contain significant deposits of iron and usually show only slight deposits in the interstitial tissue. Occasionally in cirrhosis, small quantities are found in the acinar cells.

The Bone Marrow

The bone marrow is often a rusty colour and shows intra and extracellular iron (Fig. 4.13). Iron containing macrophages can be observed in marrow smears from Black patients. In some cases there is an association between severe iron overload and osteoporosis, the bony trabeculae are smaller and more delicate than normal.

Brain and Choroid Plexus

Iron is never found in the brain substance but occasional small deposits may be found in the choroid plexus.

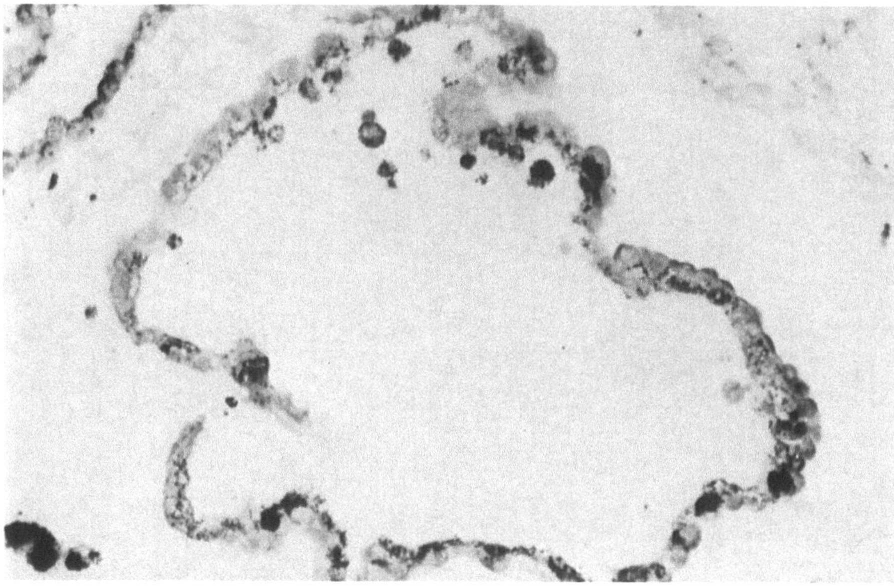

Fig. 4.14. Iron in follicular cells of thyroid. Perl's Prussian blue, ×415

Endocrine Glands

In the main, in cases of severe iron overload, the thyroid glands, pituitary gland, testes and adrenal glands show scattered haemosiderin-laden macrophages in the interstitial tissue only. In some severe cases, the endothelial cells of the sinuses of the adrenal cortex may be outlined by haemosiderin, and heavy deposits may be present in the medulla, but generally no pigment is observed in the epithelial cells. In the presence of cirrhosis, with an alteration in the distribution of iron, haemosiderin deposits may be found in the follicular cells of the thyroid (Fig. 4.14) and the epithelial cells of the pituitary and adrenal glands (Fig. 4.15). Even in the presence of cirrhosis with severe iron overload and heavy epithelial deposits throughout the body, iron in the testes is predominantly in the interstitial tissue.

Muscle

Iron deposits are rarely found in voluntary muscle and smooth muscle has not been shown to contain iron.

Lung

The lung is not a site of predilection for iron deposits and iron may be found in only small quantities in the macrophages of the interstitial tissue.

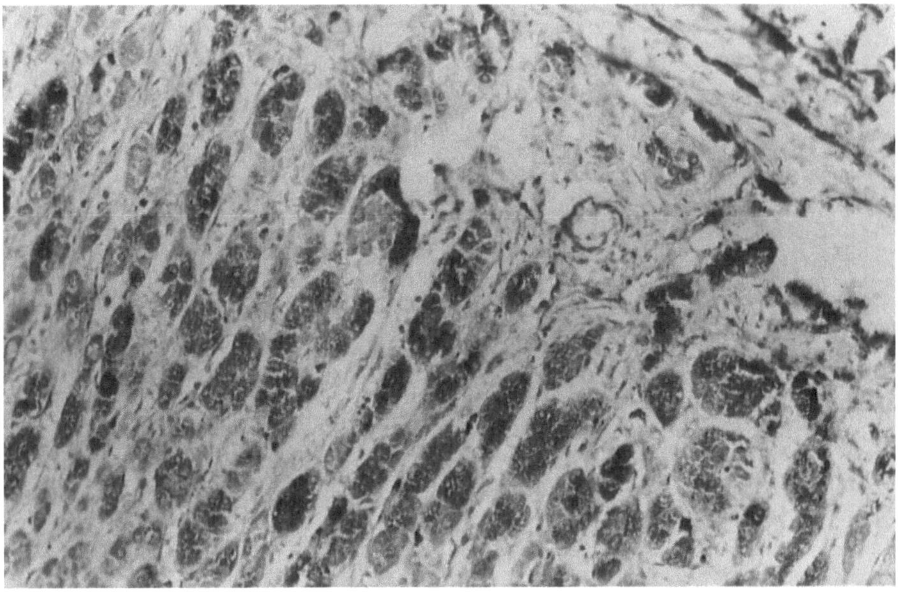

Fig. 4.15. Haemosiderin granules in the epithelial cells of the adrenal in case of iron overload with cirrhosis. The heaviest deposits are in the zona glomerulosa. Perl's Prussian blue, × 175

Higginson et al. (1953) describe two other fuchsinophilic brownish pigments present in many organs throughout the body which appear to be unrelated to the amount of haemosiderin present.

Differences Between African Siderosis and Idiopathic Haemochromatosis

The absence, in the majority of cases, of significant haemosiderin deposits in Bantu siderosis in the epithelial cells of the pancreas, stomach, thyroid, salivary and supra renal glands and the myocardium, is in striking contrast to idiopathic haemochromatosis, where these organs are almost invariably pigmented.

Pigment deposits in the jejunum and duodenum are not a feature of idiopathic haemochromatosis, where only occasional small quantities of iron are present in the villi (*Astaldi* et al. 1966). Whereas diabetes does occur in a small percentage of patients with iron overload and cirrhosis, in idiopathic haemochromatosis diabetes is present in nearly 80% of cases. Generally, in idiopathic haemochromatosis, the bone marrow contains only small quantitites of iron, whereas in African siderosis it is heavily pigmented.

The basic differentiation that has to be made is not between African siderosis as seen in the majority of subjects, and idiopathic haemochromatosis, but African siderosis associated with cirrhosis and idiopathic haemochromatosis. In the usual type of iron overloaded Black subject the distribution of iron is predominantly reticulo-endothelial, apart from the liver, whereas in idiopathic haemochromatosis the iron is essentially distributed in parenchymal cells. *Bothwell* et al. (1965) have pointed out that there are two main differences between the distribution of iron in African subjects with iron overload and cirrhosis and in White subjects with idiopathic haemochromatosis. The splenic iron concentrations are much greater in the Black patients, and in addition the distribution of iron in the liver is different. In idiopathic haemochromatosis, the major impact is on parenchymal cells with lesser amounts in Kupffer cells and bile duct epithelium and very little in portal tract phagocytes. The deposits in the African are particularly prominent in the Kupffer cells and portal tract phagocytes, with little in bile duct epithelium.

Differences Between Alcoholic Cirrhosis with Siderosis and African Siderosis with Cirrhosis

The distribution of iron and the changes in alcoholic cirrhosis with siderosis are very similar to the findings in African siderosis with cirrhosis. The quantities of iron in African siderosis are generally much greater but the distribution in both groups is very similar. This finding lends further credence to the view, that the alteration in the distribution of iron in African siderosis with cirrhosis, is more likely a result of the development of the cirrhosis than any other factor.

Transfusional Siderosis

The findings in transfusional siderosis vary somewhat from those in idiopathic haemochromatosis and African siderosis. There seem to be a number of cases with transfusional siderosis, in which iron is present in significant amounts in the parenchymal cells of organs other than the liver, in the absence of fully developed cirrhosis. As compared with idiopathic haemochromatosis, subjects with transfusional siderosis show considerably more iron in the spleen. They do not show significant cardiac involvement and most of the liver function tests are normal.

Changing Patterns of Dietary Iron Overload

Introduction

There has been a reduction in both the prevalence and severity of iron overload in urban South African Black males over the past 20 years. This can be ascribed to several radical changes in drinking habits. Firstly, commercial breweries are now the major source of fermented alcoholic drinks and very little is brewed in the home. In addition, commercially produced beers which were in the past prepared or transported in iron containers are now produced in stainless steel equipment.

Secondly, when beer is produced in the home it is usually prepared in plastic containers and not in the traditional iron drums. The third, and possibly most significant, change in the drinking habits of the urban Black population was brought about by ammendments to the liquor Act in 1961 and 1963. Prior to this the purchase of spirits by Black South Africans was prohibited. The change has resulted in a marked increase in the consumption of spirits, notably brandy and fortified wine, with a corresponding decrease in the consumption of home brewed traditional beverages.

To confirm this changing pattern of iron overload, liver specimens obtained at necropsy were studied (*MacPhail* et al. 1979).

Materials and Methods

Specimens of liver were obtained at consecutive necropsies on 248 male and 181 female adult subjects. They were fixed in buffered formal saline and the concentrations of nonheme iron were measured (*Torrance* and *Bothwell* 1968). The results were compared with those obtained in an earlier study (*Bothwell* and *Isaacson* 1962).

In addition to the chemical measurements, sections of the livers were stained for connective tissue using Masson's method and the degree of fibrosis assessed.

Results

Hepatic Iron Concentrations at Different Ages

A comparison was made between the hepatic iron concentrations in the early (1959–1960) and recent (1976) studies at different ages in the two sexes (Fig. 4.16).

In males the mean iron concentration rose with age in both groups. The mean hepatic iron concentration was lower in the 1976 group in each decade up to the age

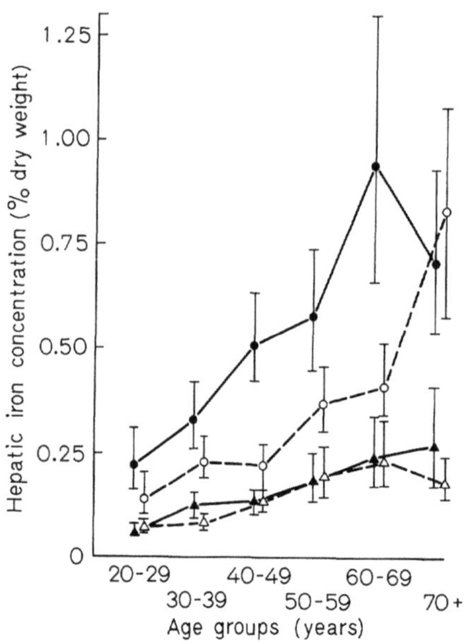

Fig. 4.16. Hepatic iron concentrations at different ages in a population measured 16 to 17 years apart. Values are geometric means (± SE). •——• Males 1959–60. ○---○ Males 1976. ▲——▲ Females 1959–60. △---△ Females 1976. (*MacPhail* et al. 1979)

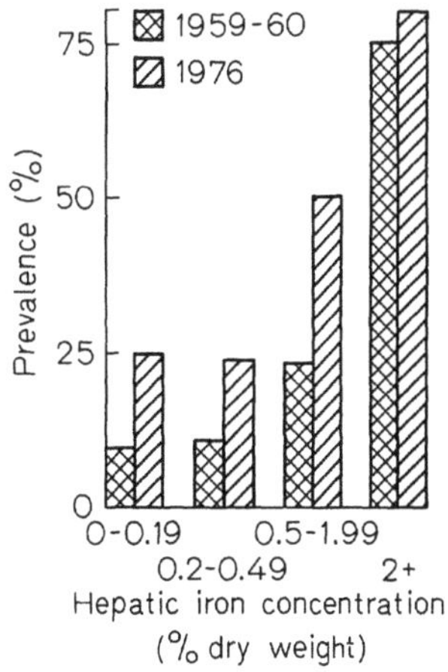

Fig. 4.17. Prevalence of portal fibrosis and cirrhosis correlated with hepatic iron concentration. Statistically significant differences ($p < 0.05$ x^2 method) between 1959–60 and 1976 groups with hepatic iron less than 2% dry weight. (*MacPhail* et al. 1979)

of 70 years. The two necropsy studies can be considered as samples of the same population taken 16 to 17 years apart. Thus the male group 40 to 49 years in the 1976 study is a sample of approximately the same population as the age group 20 to 29 years in the 1959 to 1960 study. Since the accumulation of hepatic iron is age related, the mean concentration in 1976 should be higher. The expected rise is not, however, apparent.

In females there were no significant differences between the 1959–1960 and the 1976 subjects.

Hepatic Siderosis and Portal Fibrosis

A comparison was made between the two groups with respect to the prevalence of significant portal fibrosis and cirrhosis as a function of the iron concentration (Fig. 4.17). There was a steady increase in the prevalence of significant portal fibrosis and cirrhosis with rising hepatic iron concentrations. However, portal fibrosis and cirrhosis were significantly more prevalent in the 1976 groups at all iron concentrations except those above 2% dry weight. The increased prevalence was confirmed by comparing the findings in subjects with hepatic iron concentrations less than 0.19% dry weight. Portal fibrosis and cirrhosis were present significantly more often in the 1976 study in all age groups except 40 to 49 years and above 60 years (Fig. 4.18).

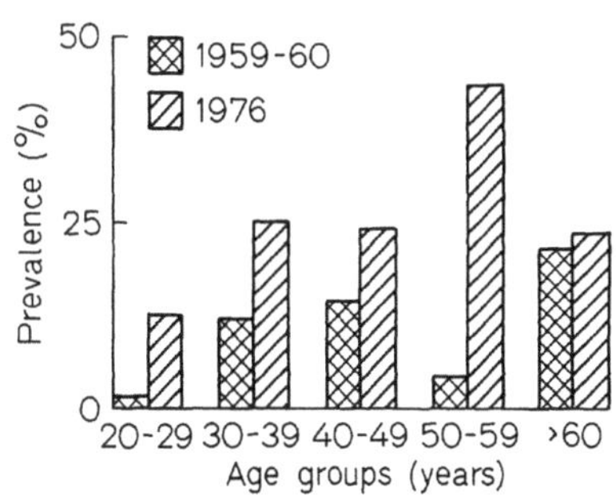

Fig. 4.18. Prevalence of portal fibrosis and cirrhosis at different ages in subjects with normal and slightly increased liver iron concentration (< 0.19% dry weight). Statistically significant differences ($p < 0.05$ x^2 method) between 1959–60 and 1976 groups at ages 20–29, 30–39 and 50–59 years. (*MacPhail* et al. 1979)

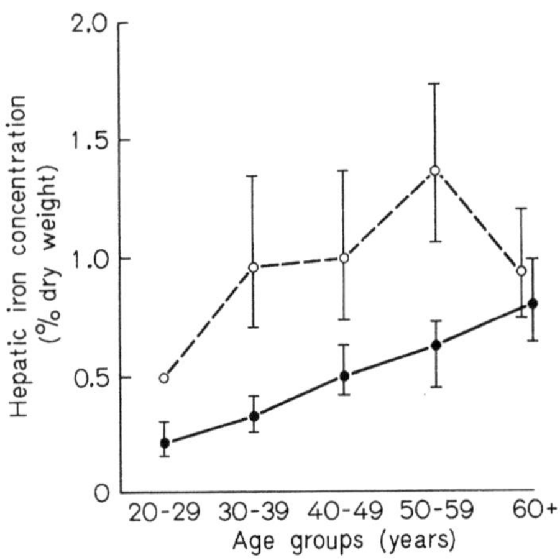

Fig. 4.19. Hepatic iron concentrations at different ages in black males who died of esophageal carcinoma compared to those who died of other causes during the same period. Values are geometric means (± SE). ○ — — ○ Esophageal carcinoma. ●——● Other causes. (*MacPhail* et al. 1979)

Carcinoma of the Esophagus

As an incidental study, the mean hepatic iron concentrations of male subjects dying of carcinoma of the esophagus were estimated and compared with the general population. The mean hepatic iron concentrations of the male subjects aged 30–39, 40–49 and 50–59 years who died of carcinoma of the esophagus between 1959 and 1964 were significantly higher than those of the males in these age groups who died of other causes in 1959–1960 (Fig. 4.19).

Discussion

This investigation confirmed a significant decrease in the prevalence of iron overload in Black male subjects dying in Baragwanath Hospital, and therefore, probably in the Black male population of Johannesburg, over the last two decades. While the prevalence of severe iron overload (hepatic iron concentration 1% dry weight) is still high (24.6%), it is significantly lower than it was previously (43.2%). In addition, there has been a corresponding, though less striking increase in the proportion of subjects with hepatic iron concentrations in the range of normal or slightly above normal. In contrast to the results in males, hepatic iron concentrations have virtually remained unchanged in females over the last 20 years.

This study also demonstrates that although the prevalence and severity of iron overload in the last 16–18 years has decreased markedly, this has been accompanied by a paradoxical increase in the prevalence of portal fibrosis and cirrhosis (Figs. 4.17, 4.18). This suggests that other factors must be at play, the most important of which is almost certainly the consumption of "The White man's liquor". It may well be that the insult of alcohol is now greater than it was in the past, since spirits and fortified wine have now replaced the traditional beverages which had an alcoholic content of only 3%. In spite of these qualifications it should however, be stressed that iron overload is still probably an important factor in the genesis of fibrotic reactions in the liver in Black adult subjects, since the highest prevalences of significant portal fibrosis or cirrhosis were noted in those subjects with hepatic iron concentrations above 2% dry weight. This was true not only in the 1959–1960 group but also in the 1976 group.

The high prevalence of carcinoma of the esophagus in adult Black subjects in South Africa is discussed in chapter 6. Although its aetiology remains obscure, it is almost certainly the result of some environmental carcinogen. The fact that the mean hepatic iron concentrations were significantly greater in subjects with carcinoma of the esophagus, and that in as many as 62% of them the values were higher than 1% dry weight, indicates a greater than average consumption of ironcontaining alcoholic beverages. However, hepatic iron concentrations were normal or only slightly raised in 13% of subjects. A possible link between iron overload and carcinoma of the esophagus is provided by the fact that ascorbic acid deficiency is extremely common in dietary iron overload (*Lynch* et al. 1967). This may make such subjects more susceptible to carcinogenic nitrosamines, since there is recent evidence that ascorbic acid inhibits the formation of N-nitroso compounds from nitrosatable amines and nitrite both in vitro and in vivo (*Mirvish* 1975).

Summary

The Blacks of Southern Africa consume a diet with a high iron content and the majority of adults at autopsy show varying degrees of siderosis. The iron is derived from iron containers used in the preparation of fermented alcoholic beverages. There is an association between severe hepatic siderosis and portal fibrosis. In most instances the iron is confined to the liver and reticulo-endothelial system, but in the presence of cirrhosis, it moves into other parenchymal cells. Most studies tend to confirm that iron has a low fibrogenic potential. Subjects with cirrhosis and iron in other parenchymal cells may develop diabetes. Over the last 17 years there has been a significant reduction in the prevalence and severity of dietary iron overload attributed to a decrease in the consumption of traditionally brewed beer.

Chapter 5

Liver Cirrhosis

Types of Cirrhosis

Higginson et al. (1957) described two major liver lesions in the adult Black of Southern Africa:

1) A diffuse portal fibrosis which, in the more severe cases, was associated with well marked siderosis (micronodular cirrhosis).

2) A "severe" cirrhosis which, in most cases, suggested to these authors a post-necrotic pathogenesis (macronodular). More than half of this group developed hepatocellular carcinoma.

The different age distribution and pathologic patterns of these two lesions suggested that they were not related. Of their 48 cases of cirrhosis 5 were of the micronodular (portal, septal) and 39 of the macronodular (postnecrotic) variety. Four were of indefinite type. The macronodular variety thus constituted over 80% of their cirrhotics. They noted that fatty change was rare in adults, but when present was often associated with tuberculosis. They found a relationship between siderosis on the one hand and fibrosis and micronodular cirrhosis on the other.

Gillman et al. (1958) and *Isaacson* et al. (1961) found a higher percentage of the micronodular type of cirrhosis. In the series of *Isaacson* et al. (1961) cirrhotics constituted 5.4% of all autopsies.

Gillman et al. (1958) also noted that fatty change associated with cirrhosis as described in European alcoholics, does not constitute a problem in adult Africans, and they also failed to find any evidence to substantiate the view that macronodular cirrhosis may be the end result of viral hepatitis. They suggested that the aetiology of macronodular cirrhosis may be related to some toxin consumed in the diet or administered by witchdoctors.

Pathology of Cirrhosis

Micronodular (Septal, Portal, Laennec's, Monolobular) Cirrhosis

Macroscopically, the liver is enlarged and weighs up to 400 g. The colour is usually brown, as most of the livers are associated with marked iron overload. The surface is finely granular due to nodules varying in size from 1–4 mm, separated by a fibrous network. The cut surface also presents a brown colour with a fine granularity. The latter may be difficult to detect macroscopically and is best viewed by slanted light (see Fig. 4.3). Microscopically, there is increased fibrosis of the portal tracts with the fibrous bands extending into the parenchyma, linking up, and thus subdividing the normal liver lobule into smaller pseudolobules. The bands of fibrous tissue vary in thickness, some being comparatively thin whereas others measure up to 600 μ. Based on the appearances in precirrhotic cases, it is apparent that the fibrous bands originate in the portal areas and radiate towards other portal tracts or towards the centre of the lobule. In the later stages, it may be impossible to assess the morphogenetic pathway of the fibrous tissue proliferation, the architecture being grossly distorted, and showing collagenous bundles containing isolated liver cells, proliferating bile ducts, inflammatory cells and blood vessels. In such areas distinction from a macronodular picture may be impossible. Proliferating, isolated liver cells may form pseudoacini resembling bile ducts. The individual liver cells generally show few abnormalities and signs of atypia are infrequent. They may be larger than normal and show cytoplasmic pallor. Mallory's alcoholic hyalin is not seen, and fatty change is infrequent, and when present of slight degree. Rarely areas of necrosis may occur distributed randomly in the lobules. The portal tracts generally contain moderate numbers of lymphocytes, and plasma cells.

The striking feature in most of these livers is the intense iron overload. Haemosiderin is present in large quantities in the hepatocytes, Kupffer cells and fibrous tissue of the portal tracts. According to *Gillman* et al. (1958) the earliest microscopic change is the appearance of fine granules of iron-containing material, primarily along the biliary poles of the liver cells, associated with only minimal amounts in the Kupffer cells. This stage is followed by aggregation within the liver cells of initially, fine, iron-containing granules into coarse lumps, and simultaneously, by the appearance of iron in significant amounts in the Kupffer cells and to varying extents in the portal phagocytes. In the later stages, masses of iron are found in clumps of phagocytes intralobularly and in the portal tracts. The centres of regenerating nodules contain less iron than the periphery. Less than 3% of all cirrhotics fall into the category of non pigmentary micronodular cirrhosis (*Wainwright* 1957). The typical microscopic appearances of micronodular cirrhosis are shown in (Figs. 5.1–5.3).

The micronodular cirrhoses are infrequently the site of hepatocellular carcinoma. In the series of *Isaacson* et al. (1961) one case out of 24 had a hepatocellular carcinoma. Because these cirrhoses are associated with heavy beer drinking, it is clear that the consumption of home-brewed alcoholic beverages does not play an aetiological role in hepatocellular carcinoma.

Macronodular (Multilobular, Postnecrotic) Cirrhosis

These livers, as the name implies are supposedly the result of large areas of necrosis undergoing collapse and scarring. The organ is therefore, grossly distorted and shows nodules from a few mm to 6 cm in diameter. The nodules are surrounded by dense bands of fibrous tissue. Foci of necrosis within individual lobules may be visible as areas of yellowish discoloration. Most livers are heavier than normal.

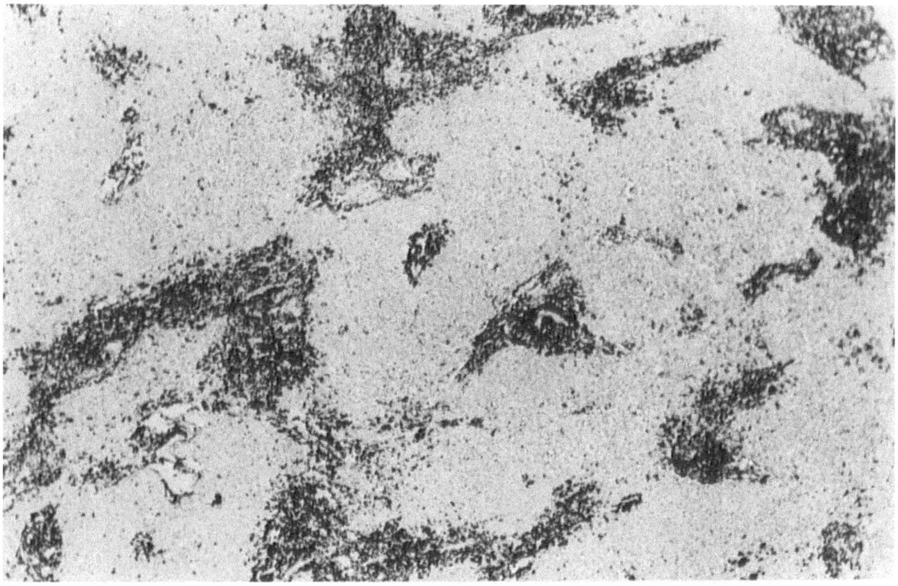

Fig. 5.1. Liver showing marked haemosiderosis with increased portal tract fibrosis but no cirrhosis. Perl's Prussian blue, × 70

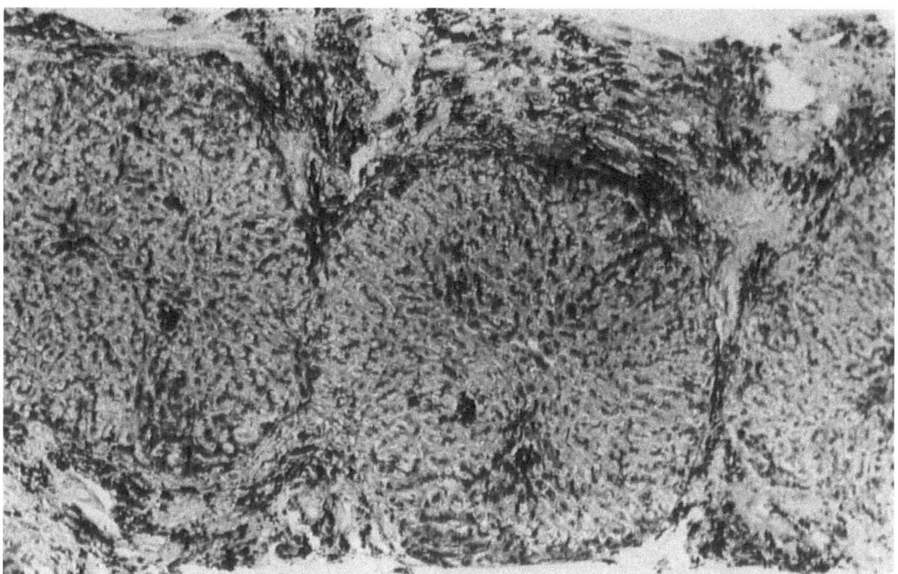

Fig. 5.2. Micronodular cirrhosis with marked iron overload. Perl's Prussian blue, × 70

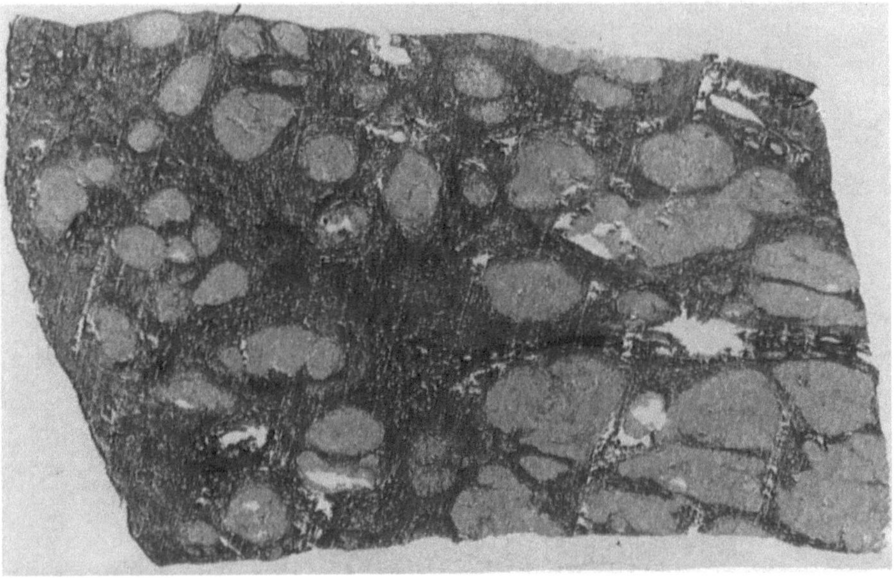

Fig. 5.3. Low power view of reticulin impregnation to show small nodules of micronodular cirrhosis. Sweets reticulin, × 12

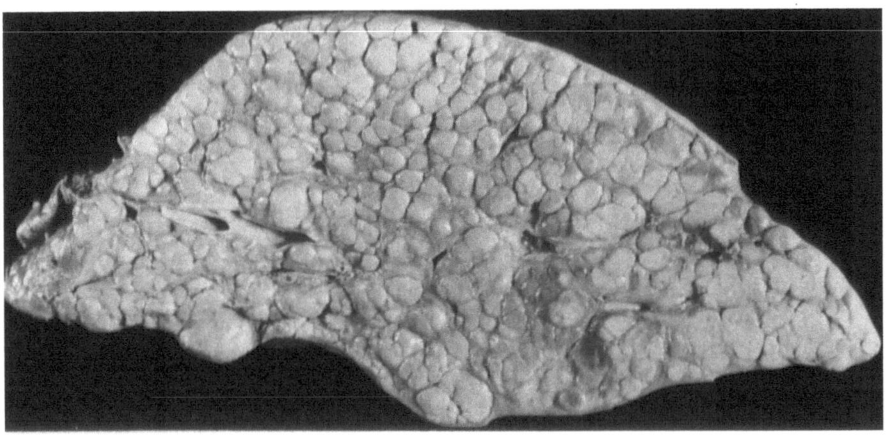

Fig. 5.4. Macroscopic appearance of macronodular cirrhosis with large regenerating nodules

Nearly one half of these cirrhotics will have developed a hepatocellular carcinoma by the time they come to autopsy. The foci of malignancy will generally appear paler than the surrounding nodules, and may be solitary or multiple (Fig. 5.4).

Microscopically, the multilobular nature of the nodules is clearly visible, most nodules consisting of two or more lobules. Many of the liver cords are two or more cells thick and the individual liver cells may be larger than normal. There may be liver

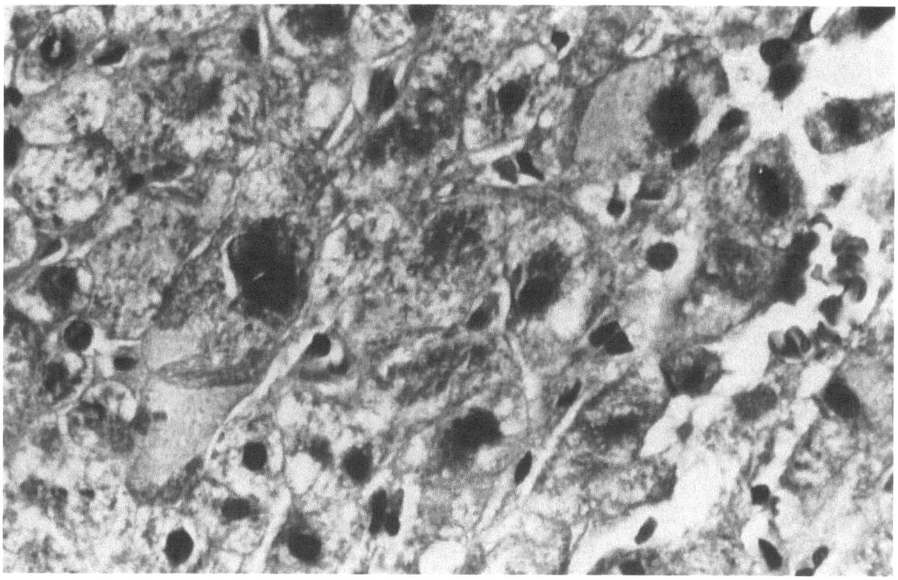

Fig. 5.5. Dysplastic liver cells in a macronodular cirrhosis, H&E, ×670

cell dysplasia with pyknotic, atypical, pleomorphic cells which may even show occasional mitoses. These findings are seldom seen in micronodular cirrhosis. As the scars are presumably preceded by necrosis and collagenization of the parenchyma, they do not arise in any particular relationship to portal tracts or central veins. Evidence of previous parenchymal collapse may be present in the apposition of three or more portal tracts.

Lymphocytes, plasma cells and scanty neutrophils are usually present in the fibrous tissue. The cirrhotic process may still be active as evidenced by foci of piecemeal necrosis, with strands of fibrous tissue surrounding small groups of necrotic liver cells. Iron overload is not a feature of this type of cirrhosis and when present is co-incidental. When a hepatocellular carcinoma is present in an iron overloaded liver, the tumour generally contains no iron. The microscopic appearances of macronodular cirrhosis are shown in (Figs. 5.5–5.8).

Aetiology of Cirrhosis

Malnutrition and Kwashiorkor

Higginson et al. (1957) thought that the age gap between the fatty liver of kwashiorkor and the development of cirrhosis in adulthood indicated that the latter was not a direct sequel of malnutrition. They did, however, suggest that damage to the liver in infancy and childhood may render the organ more susceptible to stresses in adult life. *Trowell* et al. (1954) originally stated that an appearance resembling mild Laennec's

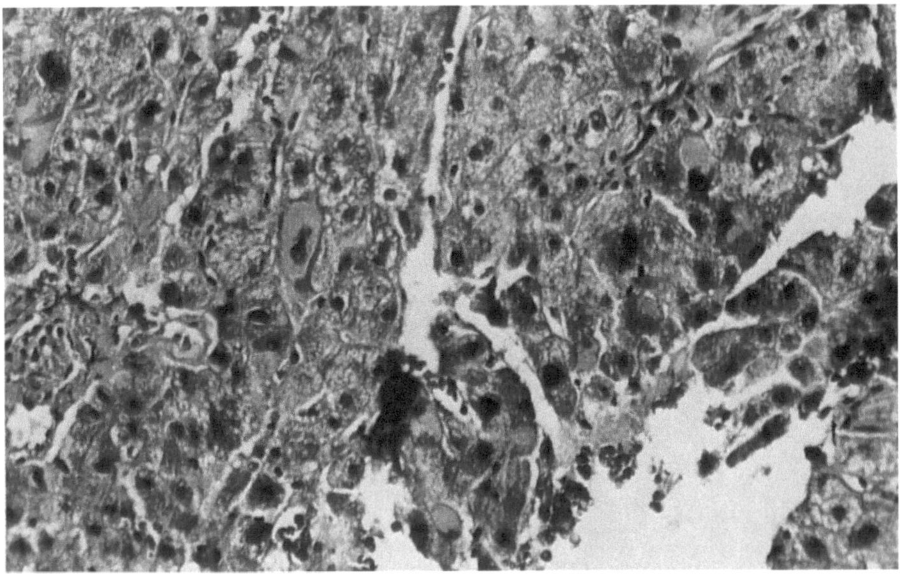

Fig. 5.6. Dysplastic hepatocytes in a macronodular cirrhosis. H&E, ×270

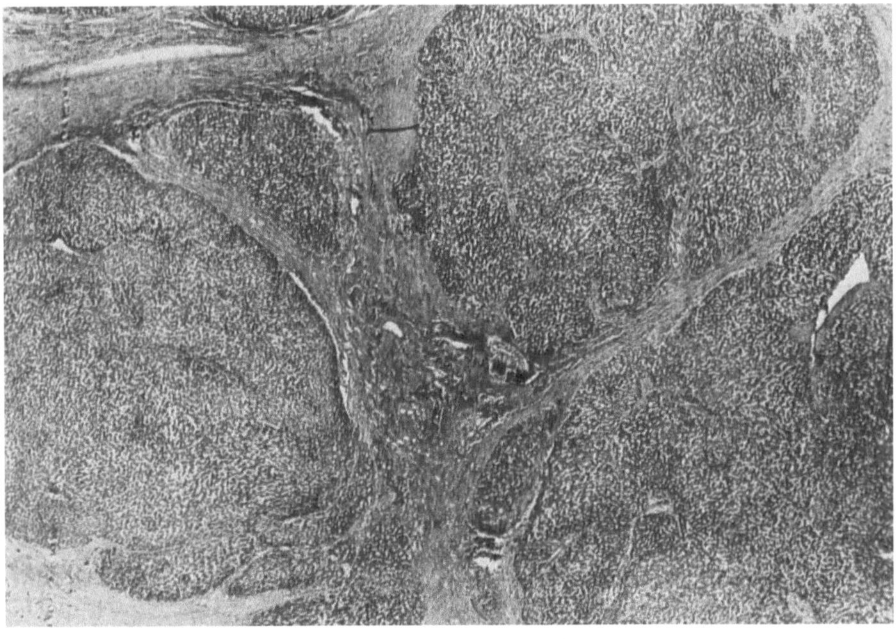

Fig. 5.7. Low power view of macronodular cirrhosis with large regenerating nodules. H&E, ×18

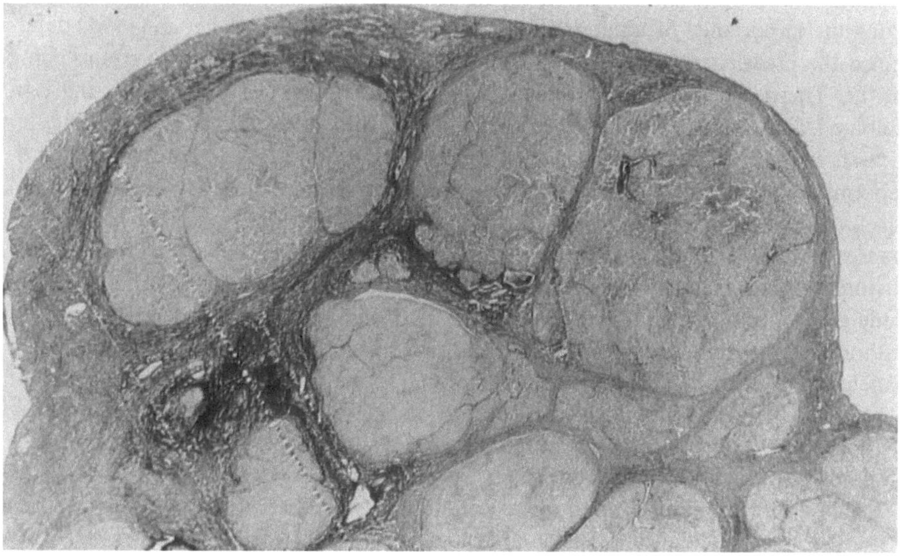

Fig. 5.8. Low power view of reticulin impregnation in a case of macronodular nodular cirrhosis. Sweets reticulin, × 10

cirrhosis may occur in older children not treated for kwashiorkor, and who have passed through the fatty liver stage for a prolonged period. The fatty liver of kwashiorkor is a true example of human liver disease due to inadequate diet, but there is no evidence that progressive fibrosis, cirrhosis or other sequelae develop directly in such livers (*Gillman* and *Gillman* 1945, 1951; *Brock* 1954; *Rhodes* 1957; *Higginson* et al. 1957; *Back* and *Bras* 1958).

Stein and *Isaacson* (1960) have shown that in childhood, in a population where protein malnutrition is common, the incidence and the causation of cirrhosis of the liver do not differ fundamentally from what is encountered in overseas populations with a vastly superior nutritional background.

Viral Hepatitis

Numerous workers have invoked viral hepatitis as a cause of the postnecrotic or macronodular cirrhosis (*Higginson* et al. 1957; *Becker* 1957; *Steiner* 1960). The absence until recently, of a satisfactory test for hepato toxic viruses, made it difficult to confirm this hypothesis.

With the recent development of histochemical, immunological and fluorescent techniques for the determination of hepatitis B virus, the picture has changed radically. *Kew* et al. (1974) examined the serum of 147 Black patients during the acute stage of hepatitis, and found hepatitis B antigen in 54% of 63 children and 65% of 83 adults. They suggested that the relative predominance of virus B hepatitis in Blacks is related to the high HBAg carrier rate in this population. The majority of patients with virus B hepatitis did not give a history of parenteral exposure to the infectious agent, emphasizing the importance of nonparenteral spread of virus B. *Bersohn* et al. (1974) determined the prevalence of hepatitis B in healthy persons of various ethnic groups living in the Transvaal, and the prevalence was 0.09–0.6% in healthy Whites, 0.9% in Coloured donors, 2% in urban Negroes, and 7% in rural male Blacks. Their findings indicated that geographical environment might be one of the factors influencing antigenaemia in healthy persons and that antigenaemia was three times as common in rural Black subjects as in urban persons of similar tribal origin. The high incidence in rural areas may be due to the scarification which is frequently practised as part of the tribal customs. As the majority of hepatocellular carcinomas arise in livers the site of macronodular cirrhosis, the study of *Macnab* et al. (1976) is of extreme interest. These authors investigating the presence of hepatitis B surface antigen and antibody in Black patients with primary hepatocellular carcinoma, found surface antigen in the serum of 58 of 158 (36.4%) by immunoelectrophoresis and in 94 (59.5%) by radio immune assay (RIA). The prevalence of this antigen in the general Black population using these methods was 7% and 9% respectively.

Many authors have claimed an association between hepatitis B virus on the one hand and macronodular cirrhosis and hepatocellular carcinoma on the other (*Maynard* et al. 1970; *Sherlock* et al. 1970; *Vogel* et al. 1970; *Anthony* 1972; *Kew* et al. 1974). In the series of *Kew* et al. (1974) macronodular cirrhosis was present in 60% of their subjects with hepatocellular carcinoma, and HBAg was not found significantly more often in these patients than in those without cirrhosis. Nor was cirrhosis encountered significantly more frequently in patients with antigenaemia than in those without. These observations suggest that if primary liver cancer is a consequence of the persistence of hepatitis virus, the latter must be directly oncogenic, in addition to having the potential to induce neoplasia indirectly via chronic parenchymal liver disease.

Alternatively, their findings may indicate that persistence of the virus is the result and not the cause of primary liver cancer, or that some immunologic defect is responsible for both.

Primack et al. (1973) were unable to find any obvious immunologic deficiency in Ugandan patients with primary liver cancer. *Kew* et al. (1974) point out that the fact that primary liver cancer occurs commonly in some populations in which the HBAg carrier state is infrequent and virus B hepatitis not endemic and visa versa, and the far greater incidence of this tumour in males, indicates that persistence of the hepatitis B virus is not the only aetiological factor in primary liver cancer. They suggest that it may act in conjunction with other toxic, nutritional or hormonal factors to induce neoplastic change. Their failure to elicit a history of a hepatitis-like illness is similar to the experience in Taiwan (*Tong* et al. 1971) and Uganda (*Vogel* et al. 1970), and this may reflect the frequency with which virus B hepatitis is clinically mild and anicteric. Countries in which primary liver cancer is rare e.g. the United States show no obvious relationship between chronic HBAg antigenaemia and hepatocellular carcinoma, indicating that other factors must also be involved in the aetiology (*Macnab* et al. 1976).

There are countries with a high carrier rare of the virus and a high prevalence of chronic liver disease associated with HBAg antigenaemia with a low incidence of primary liver cancer, suggesting that the virus may only be oncogenic in combination with one or more other factors (*Theodoropoulos* et al. 1975). Dysplasia of liver cells tends to be associated with the presence of HBAg (*Anthony* 1972).

Toxins

A toxin may be the underlying aetiological factor in some cases of cirrhosis. Many Blacks still seek treatment from witchdoctors, often before coming to hospital and they are therefore exposed to a wide variety of tribal medicines, the composition and effects of which are generally unknown. *Grusin* (1955) described five cases of liver poisoning and renal failure due to potassium dichromate, a drug employed as an emetic by witchdoctors. The effect is usually massive hepatic necrosis with renal tubular necrosis. *Neame* and *Pillay* (1964) reported 11 patients with spontaneous hypoglycaemia and hepatic and renal necrosis following the intake of herbal medicines. At necropsy, there was diffuse centrilobular zonal necrosis of the liver, and renal tubular necrosis. Herbal medicine obtained in two instances and injected intraperitoneally into rats produced typical hepatic and renal lesions. Cases of liver necrosis due to the plant Callilepis laureola are well known (*Wainwright* and *Schonland* 1977). The livers at necropsy are pale and yellow with sharply demarcated centrilobular punctate congested areas, and microscopically, there are well demarcated foci of centrilobular necrosis. The peripheral hepatocytes contained abundant small fat vacuoles and inflammatory cell infiltration is minimal. The kidneys consistently show evidence of tubular necrosis, involving both the convoluted tubules and loops of Henle and hyaline, granular and red cell casts are present. No evidence however, exists that these cases progress to cirrhosis.

Aflatoxin

The comments in relation to the possible aetiological role of aflatoxin in the genesis of hepatocellular carcinoma apply equally to macronodular cirrhosis. *Oettle* (1965) suggested that the hypothesis of myocotoxicosis resulting from spoilage of food by toxic moulds fits the distribution of hepatocellular carcinoma better than any other theory, and that it accounts for the rarity of liver cancer in dry areas where mould spoilage is minimal, or in tribes, for example, in Uganda which consume a predominantly fresh diet (*Butler* 1964; *Isaacson* 1966). *Van Rensberg* et al. (1974) working in Mozambique in an area with the highest known liver cancer incidence in the world, found that the diet contains the highest known aflatoxin intake, the average adult consuming 15.6 mg of aflatoxin per day. The incidence rate of liver cell carcinoma in this area is 25.5 per 100.000 per year. Reports of toxic hepatitis possibly due to aflatoxin have emanated from Mozambique (*Torres* et al. 1970). Macronodular cirrhosis followed in some cases and in three subjects primary liver cancer supervened. Following the observation of *Peers* and *Linsell* (1973) of a significant association between liver cancer and ingested aflatoxin in a study in the Murango district of Kenya, *Bagshawe* et al. (1975) studied the incidence of hepatitis B antigen in the same district, and showed no significant difference between the low altitude area with a relatively high incidence of primary liver cancer, and the high altitude area with a lower incidence of the tumour. They concluded that current evidence favours aflatoxin playing an important role in the aetiology of primary liver cancer with hepatitis B fulfilling an ancillary function.

Sixty percent of patients with primary liver cancer have a macronodular cirrhosis (*Kew* et al. 1974), but in other parts of Africa, such as Mozambique, up to 60% of liver cell carcinomas develop in non-cirrhotic livers. Cirrhosis cannot therefore, be an essential prerequisite to cancer, as indeed it is not in the experimental animal. It seems therefore, that whatever the hepatotoxic or carcinogenic factors involved in liver disease these substances may produce hepatocellular carcinomas in livers the site of macronodular cirrhosis (between 60 and 80% of all tumours), or alternatively effect a direct oncogenic action on the liver cells producing carcinomas in the absence of cirrhosis.

A single aetiological agent could not account for all the aspects of macronodular cirrhosis and hepatocellular carcinoma in Blacks, and a likely hypothesis would implicate mycotoxins and hepatitis B virus.

Iron

Comments on the fibrogenic effect of excessive iron made in the chapter on iron overload, apply similarly to the effect of iron in the production of micronodular cirrhosis (*Higginson* et al. 1953; *Bothwell* and *Isaacson* 1962). There has been considerable dispute as to whether iron overload plays a part in the aetiology of cirrhosis (*Higginson* et al. 1953; *Higginson* et al. 1957; *Bothwell* and *Bradlow* 1960; *Bothwell* and *Isaacson* 1962). Most authors accept that there is an association between iron overload and portal tract fibrosis. Iron overload plays a significant role in the pathogenesis of micronodular cirrhosis (*Seftel* et al. 1960). If iron is not the cause of cirrhosis, it probably potentiates the effect of some other exotoxin. The source of the latter may also be alcoholic beverages. These drinks often contain other deleterious substances including carbide and cantharides. In the study by *Isaacson* et al. (1961) no association was found between siderosis and macronodular cirrhosis. This is of considerable significance in view of the fact that when a hepatocellular carcinoma arises in a cirrhotic liver, the cirrhosis is usually macronodular in type. As the iron is derived in the main from homemade alcoholic brews, this would indicate, that neither iron overload nor alcohol play a role in the aetiology of hepatocellular carcinoma. If a toxin is responsible for the development of macronodular cirrhosis and hepatocellular carcinoma it is unlikely to be found in the traditional alcoholic beverages.

For further discussion of the role of iron in liver disease – refer to Chapter 4.

Liver Disease in Children

Cirrhosis in Children

For many years it was believed that the fatty liver of kwashiorkor may progress to cirrhosis (*Waterlow* 1948; *Trowell* et al. 1954). However, most later workers found that portal fibrosis was not a direct sequel of kwashiorkor (*Gillman* and *Gillman* 1951; *Brock* 1954; *Higginson* et al. 1957; *Rhodes* 1957; *Back* and *Bras* 1958). *Stein* and

Isaacson (1960) stated that in a child population where protein malnutrition is common, the incidence and the causation of cirrhosis of the liver do not differ fundamentally from those encountered in overseas populations with a vastly superior nutritional background. Subjects with kwashiorkor invariably show fatty infiltration of the liver but, no case has been encountered where this was associated with cirrhosis. Mild periportal fibrosis with increased reticulin is found in the livers of malnourished children, but there is never any architectural distortion of the liver lobule or regenerative hyperplasia. Thus while it is possible that the fatty liver of kwashiorkor may render the adult liver in later life more susceptible to other hepatotoxic agents, the view that kwashiorkor progresses directly to cirrhosis, is quite untenable. Children with kwashiorkor and hepatic steatosis either recover completely or die.

At Baragwanath Hospital 2 to 3 cases of congenital extra hepatic obliteration of the bile ducts are admitted annually. Neonatal hepatitis is fairly common, about 6–8 cases being diagnosed annually. No examples of cirrhosis due to glycogen storage disease of the liver or galactosaemia have yet been described in Blacks. Cardiac cirrhosis has not been found. Bilharzia is of no significance in the pathogenesis of cirrhosis in Black children. Positive serology for syphilis is not uncommonly found in the mothers of children, but clinical manifestations of congenital syphilis are uncommon.

Veno-Occlusive Disease of the Liver in Black Children

The first report of veno-occlusive disease of the liver in Black African children was by *Stein* (1957) who described 3 cases. This disease is characterized by occlusion of the smaller branches of the hepatic veins, due to an endophlebitis. In the early stages, the intimal thickening is predominantly due to oedema, but later is due to connective tissue proliferation. The venous obstruction produced by the endophlebitis of the central hepatic veins, results in centrilobular congestion and rupture of the sinusoids to form centrilobular blood lakes, with necrosis of adjacent hepatocytes. Patients may recover from this stage or progress to the subacute stage and ultimately cirrhosis. Clinically, the acute phase manifests itself with the sudden onset of ascites and hepatomegaly. The original description of this disease in humans was by *Selzer* and *Parker* (1951) who reported 12 cases in White and Coloured adults and children, and suggested that the condition was caused by the consumption of bread made of inadequately winnoed wheat, and contaminated with senecio or ragwort, a common wild plant. The majority of cases of veno-occlusive disease have been reported from Jamaica (*Jellife* et al. 1957; *Hill* et al. 1958). The disease has three clinical and histological phases the acute phase having an abrupt onset, with hepatomegaly and ascites and the liver at this stage showing intense centrilobular congestion with oedematous endophlebitis of the smaller branches of the hepatic veins (Figs. 5.9, 5.10). There may be recovery from this stage, or progression to the subacute phase with persistent hepatomegaly, which may also be associated with ascites, and during this phase, the central veins of the liver are blocked by a fibrous endophlebitis, causing further centrilobular congestion with necrosis of liver cells, and this may progress to cirrhosis. The disease is believed to be caused by ingestion of the senecio group of alkaloids, and in Jamaica these occur in infusions of plants which are drunk as bush teas.

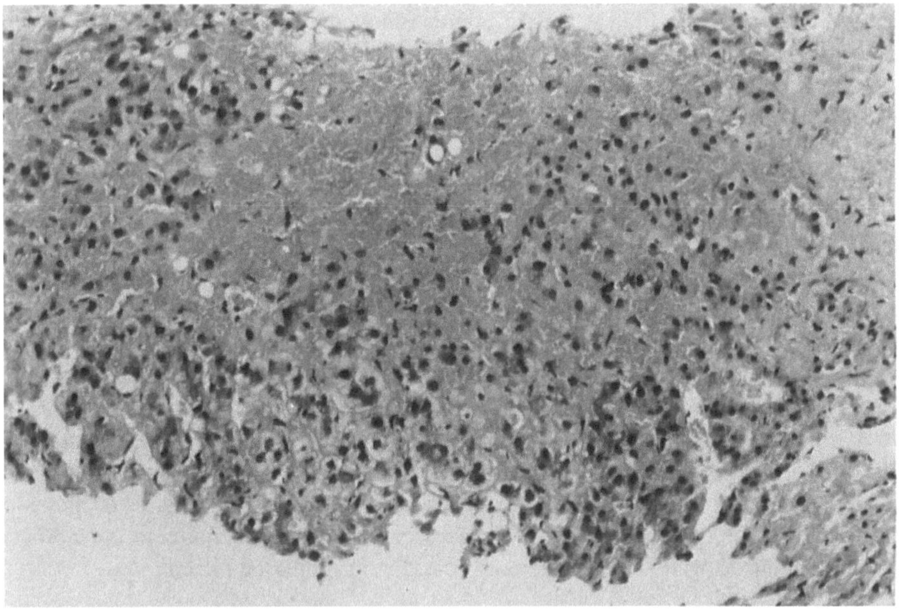

Fig. 5.9. Marked centrilobular congestion in veno-occlusive disease. The extravasated blood has produced necrosis of surrounding hepatocytes. H&E, ×175

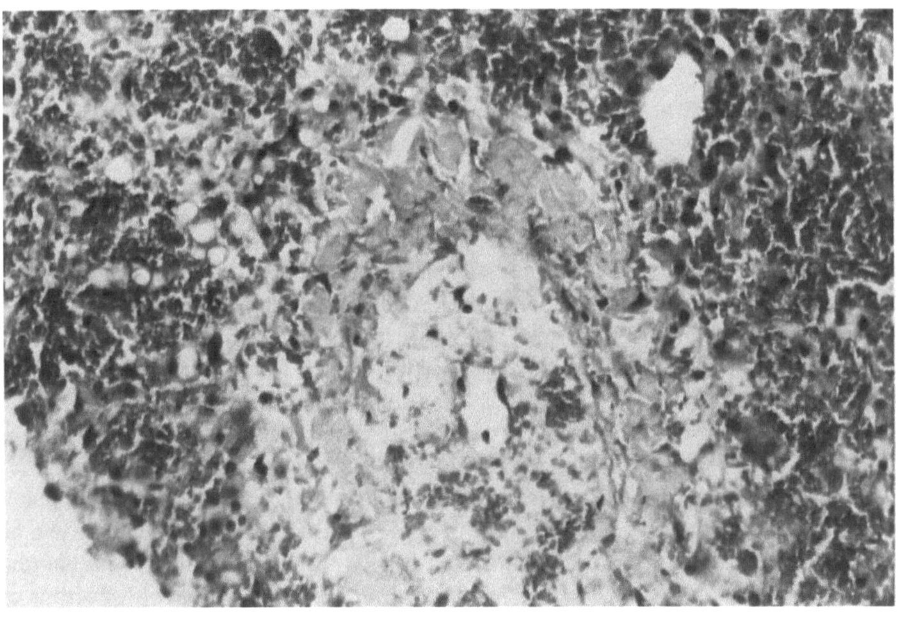

Fig. 5.10. Endophlebitis of central vein in veno-occlusive disease. H&E, ×280

Experimental veno-occlusive disease has been produced by feeding calves with crotalaria furva (*Berry* and *Bras* 1957; *Hill* et al. 1958). In the series reported by *Stein* and *Isaacson* (1962) there was no sex predilection, five of the children were less than 18 months of age, and the remaining four were between 18 months and three years. Malnutrition does not appear to be an aetiological factor and the younger the child, the poorer the prognosis. A raised serum bilirubin level is indicative of a poor prognosis.

The Changing Pattern of Liver Disease in Blacks

Introduction

Until 1962 South African Blacks were not permitted access to the usual sources of alcohol and obtained alcohol from home-brewed beverages prepared in rusting metallic containers. As described previously, this alcohol contains large quantities of iron and its consumption produces iron overload in the Black population. Micronodular cirrhosis is associated with iron overload and the consumption of large quantitiites of iron containing alcohol. This cirrhosis, characterized by the presence of large quantities of haemosiderin, until recently showed a complete absence of fatty change, alcoholic hepatitis, alcoholic hyalin or alcoholic cirrhosis. This is in contrast to the picture seen in Western societies after prolonged consumption of hard liquor. In 1962 South African Blacks were granted access to all varieties of liquor. This change in drinking habits has produced an alteration in the picture of liver disease with the appearance of micronodular cirrhosis with fatty change, alcoholic hyalin, alcoholic hepatitis and alcoholic cirrhosis (*Isaacson* 1978).

Materials and Methods

All the liver biopsy specimens received in the Baragwanath histopathology laboratory in 1959–1960 and 1975–1976 were reviewed. The criteria for performing a biopsy were the same in 1975–1976 as in 1959–1960, namely a clinical suspicion of liver disease. The material was therefore unselected and was not derived from patients giving a history of alcoholism only. As the clinical records were generally either incomplete or unavailable, the study conducted was predominantly based on pathological findings. Biopsy specimens from subjects under the age of 20 years were excluded because the pattern of liver disease in children had clearly not changed. All sections were stained with haemotoxylin and eosin, Perls's Prussian blue reaction for iron, elastic Masson and a reticulin impregnation.

Table 5.1. Comparison of liver biopsies from 1959–1960 with 1975–1976 (*Isaacson* 1978)

	1959–1960 Males	Females	Total	1975–1976 Males	Females	Total
Total	143	58	201	516	213	729
No cirrhosis no tumour	100	32	132	273	112	385
Iron +++ no cirrhosis no tumour	87	23	110	126	16	142
Micronodular cirrhosis	22	21	43	134	68	202
Iron in micronodular cirrhosis	100%	100%	100%	63%	57%	60%
Fatty change in micronodular cirrhosis	13%	9.5%	12%	34%	47%	40%
Typical alcoholic cirrhosis	0	0	0	4.4%	4.4%	4.4%
Alcoholic hyalin	0	0	0	3.7%	12%	7%
Macronodular cirrhosis	9	3	12	58	21	79
Hepatocellular carcinoma	19	3	22	68	9	77
Total number of biopsies			6287			13786

Results

The laboratory received 6278 surgical specimens during the years 1959–1960 and included in these were 201 liver biopsy specimens (148 from males and 58 from females). One hundred and thirty-two of the liver specimens did not show cirrhosis or tumour; of these, 110 (83%) showed moderate to marked iron overload. This marked degree of iron overload reflects the heavy consumption of iron-laden home-brewed alcoholic beverages. During the period 1975–1976 the laboratory received 13 786 specimens and these included 729 liver biopsy specimens (516 from males and 213 from females). Three hundred and eighty-five of these specimens did not show cirrhosis or tumour, and of these, only 142 (37%) showed moderate to marked iron overload, as compared with the 83% of the earlier series (Table 5.1).

In the 1959–1960 series there were 43 cases of micronodular cirrhosis, all of which showed heavy iron overload, with minimal fatty change in only 5. Alcoholic cirrhosis and alcoholic hyalin were not seen. In the 1975–1976 series there were 202 cases of micronodular cirrhosis, of which 124 (61%) were associated with heavy iron overload. Prominent fatty change associated with iron overload was found in 77 (38%) of the 202 cases, and 9 cases showed typical alcoholic cirrhosis. Thirteen subjects had alcoholic hyalin. One hundred and fifty-six (63%) of the patients with micronodular cirrhosis were males and the disease occurred predominantly in patients over 40 years of age (Table 5.2).

These findings demonstrate that significant fatty change and alcoholic hyalin made their appearance in the liver of Black alcoholics after the liberalization of the liquor laws and are presumably a consequence of consuming the 'White man's alcohol'. It is impossible on the basis of these figures to assess whether there has been an increase in the incidence of cirrhosis in this population, as the marked rise in the number of patients with cirrhosis over the years could reflect the increase in the number of admissions to the hospital.

Table 5.2. Cirrhosis in South African Blacks (*Isaacson* 1978)

Age (years)	1959–1960 Males		Females		1975–1976 Males		Females		Total Micro		Macro	
	Micro	Macro	Micro	Macro	Micro	Macro	Micro	Macro	M	F	M	F
20–29	1	1	0	1	3	1	1	3	4	1	2	4
30–39	6	4	3	0	7	12	7	2	13	10	16	2
40–49	5	2	6	1	16	9	11	5	21	17	11	6
50–59	4	0	3	0	36	10	14	3	40	17	10	3
60 plus	1	0	3	0	36	10	18	4	37	21	10	4
Unknown	5	2	6	1	36	16	17	4	41	23	18	5
Total	22	9	21	3	134	58	68	21	156	89	67	24
Number with hepatocellular carcinoma	4	3	2	0	2	16	1	2	6	3	19	2

Micro Micronodular cirrhosis; *Macro* macronodular cirrhosis

In the 1959–1960 series there were 12 cases of macronodular cirrhosis (9 in males), none of which showed any evidence of significant iron overload. The 1975–1976 series included 79 cases of macronodular cirrhosis (58 in males) of which 3 (all in males) showed iron overload. These findings confirm that there is no relationship between alcohol consumption, iron overload and macronodular cirrhosis (*Isaacson* et al. 1961). Macronodular cirrhosis occurred at all ages but the incidence was high from the third decade onwards (Table 5.2). Twenty-one (23%) of the patients with macronodular cirrhosis had an associated hepatocellular carcinoma. This is not an accurate reflection of the incidence of hepatocellular carcinoma in macronodular cirrhosis, because needle biopsy may not always sample the tumour. At autopsy nearly half the patients with macronodular cirrhosis have an associated hepatocellular carcinoma.

In this study there were 99 hepatocellular carcinomas (87 males) of which 22 were derived from the 1959–1960 series and 77 from the 1975–1976 series. There is no evidence of a fall in the incidence of hepatocellular carcinoma at Baragwanath Hospital. Some authors (*Harington* et al. 1975; *Bradshaw* and *Harington* 1976) claim a fall in the incidence of hepatocellular carcinoma in Shangaan miners from Mozambique working on the gold mines in South Africa.

The change in drinking habits of South African Blacks has produced an alteration in the picture of liver disease, with the appearance in micronodular cirrhosis of fatty change, alcoholic hyalin, alcoholic hepatitis and alcoholic cirrhosis. Many livers show a mixed picture of iron overload and fatty change with alcoholic hyalin, indicating consumption of traditional home-brewed beverages plus hard liquor. Alcoholic hyalin is associated with prolonged consumption of hard liquor (*Christoffersen* et al. 1973). Several cases in the 1975–1976 series showed alcoholic cirrhosis with no iron, indicating that these subjects were not consuming the traditional alcoholic beverages, but were drinking iron-free liquor only. *MacPhail* et al. (1979) have already shown that with the change in the drinking habits there has been a dramatic fall in the iron content of the livers of adult Blacks, but this has been associated with a significant rise in the incidence of portal tract fibrosis and micronodular cirrhosis suggesting that as a fibrogenic or cirrhotogenic agent, the "White man's liquor" may be more potent than traditional beer. In Western societies nearly one third of alcoholic cirrhoses show a hepatocellular carcinoma at autopsy (*Lee* 1966). With the introduction of hard liquor to the drinking habits of the Blacks it may well be that whatever the other aetiological factors in the pathogenesis of hepatocellular carcinoma, and these include mycotoxins and hepatitis B virus, an additional carcinogen in the form of the "White man's liquor" may dramatically raise the already high incidence of this tumours. Figures 5.11–5.14 depict the changing pattern of liver disease in Blacks.

Summary

Cirrhosis in this population can be divided into the two main categories of macronodular and micronodular. The micronodular is generally associated with iron overload, but does not show other features of alcoholic cirrhosis. These livers are rarely complicated by hepatocellular carcinoma. Macronodular cirrhosis on the other hand does not show significant iron overload and is frequently the site of a hepatocellular carcinoma.

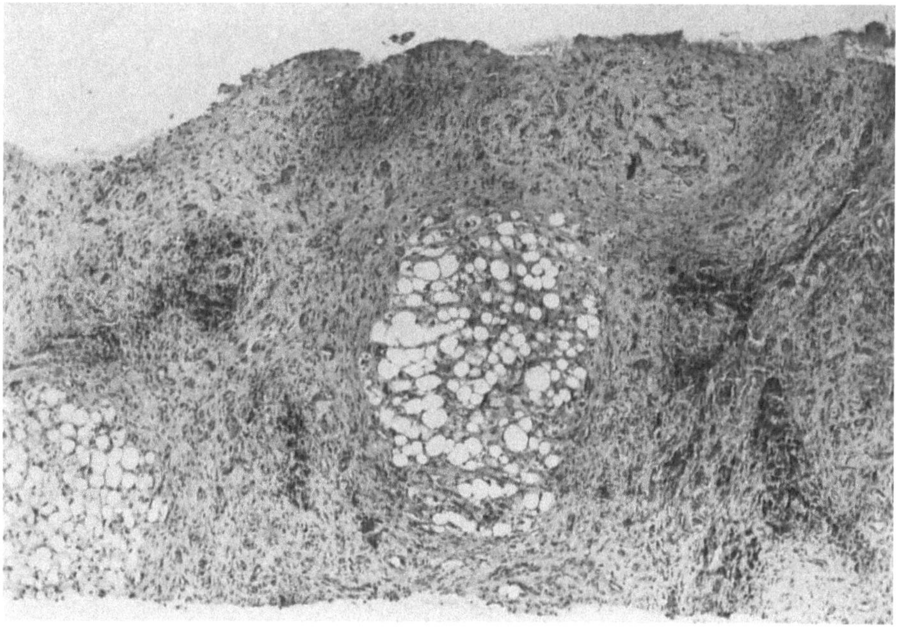

Fig. 5.11. Low power view of micronodular cirrhosis with iron overload and fatty change. H&E, × 70

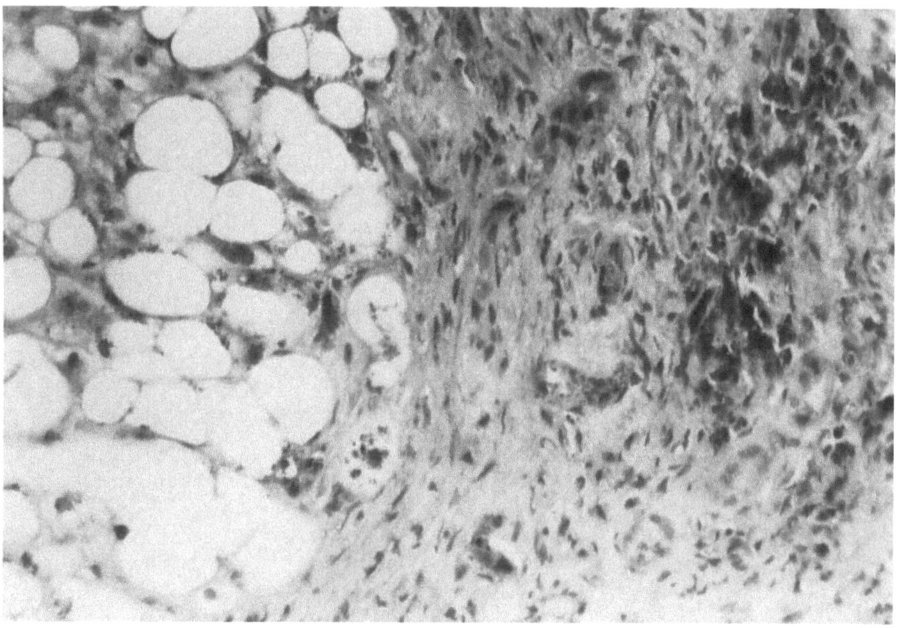

Fig. 5.12. High power of micronodular cirrhosis with iron overload and fatty change. H&E, × 290

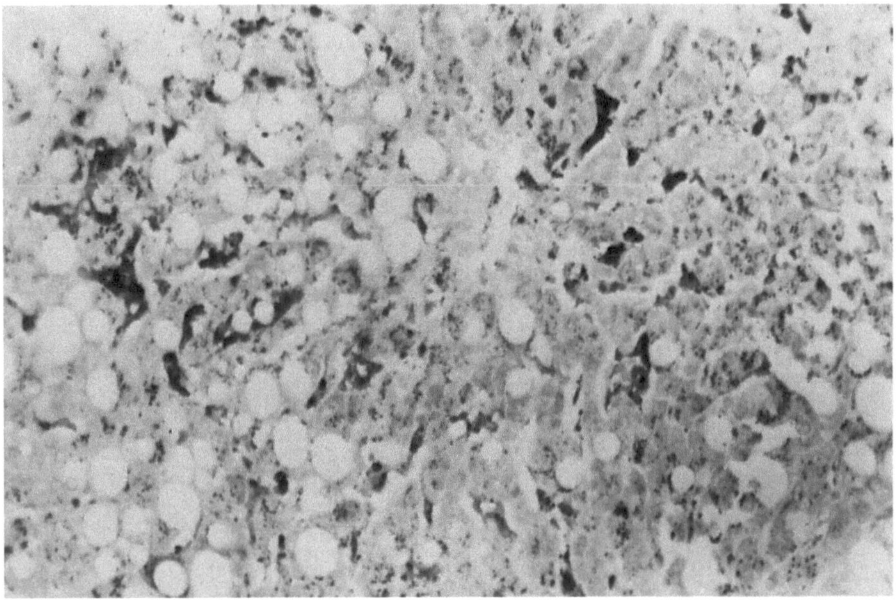

Fig. 5.13. Mixed picture of fatty change and iron overload. Perl's Prussian blue, ×280

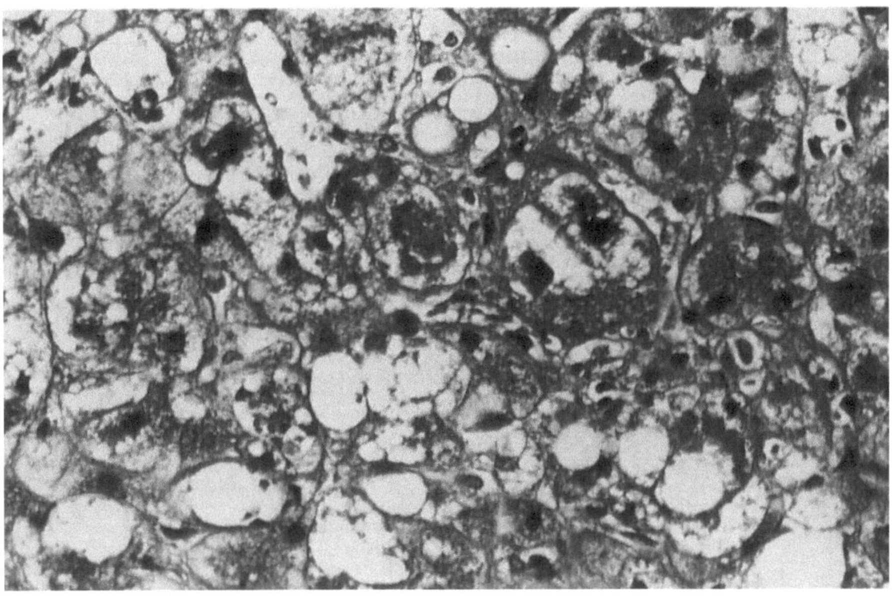

Fig. 5.14. Marked fatty change with alcoholic hyalin. H&E, ×400

The aetiology of the macronodular cirrhosis and hepatocellular carcinoma is probably multifactorial with hepatitis B and aflatoxin being important. Cirrhosis in children is not more frequent in this population than in equivalent Caucasian peoples. In recent years with the change in the type of alcohol consumed by the Black population, there has been a marked alteration in the pattern of liver disease with the development of the characteristic Western type alcoholic cirrhosis with fatty change, alcoholic hepatitis and alcoholic hyalin.

Note Added in Proof

More recent work from South Africa lends even greater weight to the oncogenic role of hepatitis B virus (*Kew* et al. 1979, 1980; *Kew* 1981). *Shafritz* and *Kew* (1981) have shown that integration of HBV-DNA into the host genome occurs in conjunction with malignant transformation. Their data suggested that integration HBV-DNA into hepatocytes occurs during the course of persistent HBV infection and precedes development of gross neoplasm (*Shafritz* et al. 1981).

Isaacson et al. (1979) examined two groups of hepatocellular carcinomas for the presence of hepatitis B surface antigen. The one was derived from the autopsy material at Baragwanath Hospital on subjects who had lived in Soweto, a large Black urban town. The second group consisted of male Black mine workers generally originating from rural areas. The two groups showed totally different results. The Baragwanath series consisted of 24 hepatocellular carcinomas of which only 17% were HBSAg positive. The series of male black mine workers comprised 22 cases of which 72% were HBSAg positive. These findings delineate two different populations of hepatocellular carcinoma in Southern Africa.

Very recently *Paterson* and *Isaacson* (1982) studied the impact of urbanisation on the relationship of hepatitis B virus to hepatocellular carcinoma. They studied cases during the period 1956–1960 and 1976–1980 and found evidence of a significant increase in overall average age in the proportion of female cases while the percentage of HBSAg positive cases had fallen.

Chapter 6

Cancer Epidemiology

Introduction

The life style of the urban Black community is changing rapidly, and the long term effects that this may have on cancer incidence is uncertain. They are discarding traditional foodstuffs in favour of White eating and drinking patterns. There has been a marked decrease in proportionate expenditure on mealie-meal, and sorghum beer, and commanding a bigger slice of income are meat, vegetables, fruits, white bread, malt beer. According to a report of the University of South Africa's Bureau of Market Research 37.5% of the expenditure on grain products was accounted for by mealie-meal in 1970, whereas the figure in 1975 was 23.5%. On the other hand the figure for White bread rose from 23% to 30.9%.

The last significant survey of cancer in the Blacks of South Africa was that by *Higginson* and *Oettle* (1960) which covered the period 1953–1955. It was considered that a survey over a longer period and using the extensive material that had accumulated in the laboratory at the same hospital would be of value (*Isaacson* et al. 1978).

Material and Methods

Baragwanath is a large (2500 bed) general hospital for Black patients. It is situated on the outskirts of Soweto, a town of approximately one million inhabitants 10 miles south west of Johannesburg. Baragwanath is the only major hospital serving the population of Soweto and it is a reasonable assumption that probably 90% of patients with malignant disease will present themselves at the hospital (*Higginson* and *Oettle* 1960). An assessment of the size of the population of Soweto is fraught with difficulties. However, an approximation was one million at about the halfway stage of the survey – 1970.

The population base of this study was therefore the actual one. The survey extended over the years 1966 to 1975. The age distribution of this population is available and thus age specific incidence rates could be computed. It was calculated that 2.5% is the approximate annual population growth and the population for each year from 1966 to 1975 was calculated by either adding or subtracting 2.5% of one million (the population in 1970). The age specific rates were calculated by adding the rates for two five year age groups, e.g., 30–34 and 35–39 and then dividing the sum by two. Statistically this is not strictly permissible, but the error so incurred is small. Ten years of cancer records from the laboratory at Baragwanath hospital were examined.

Table 6.1. Average annual incidence per 100,000 – all ages – Soweto Blacks

	Males		Females
Squamous carcinoma of the tongue	2.3		0.2
Squamous carcinoma of cheek and mouth	1.8		0.1
Salivary gland tumours (males and females)	–	1.4	
Squamous carcinoma of the oesophagus	23.7		4.2
Hepatocellular carcinoma	4.8		0.8
Squamous carcinoma of the stomach	1.7		0.5
Carcinoma of the rectum	0.7		0.7
Carcinoma of the colon	0.9		0.3
Squamous carcinoma of the antrum	2.2		0.6
Squamous carcinoma of the larynx	3.7		0.2
Carcinoma of the breast (females)	–		6.0
Squamous carcinoma of the cervix	–		19.3
Carcinoma of the endometrium	–		1.3
Chorionepithelioma	–		0.2
Tumours of the ovary	–		6.1
Carcinoma of the prostate	4.5		–
Tumours of the testis	0.2		–
Squamous carcinoma of the penis	1.3		–
Malignant tumours of the kidney (males and females)	–	0.6	–
Carcinoma of the bladder	1.2		0.3
Malignant melanoma of the skin	0.8		0.9
Tumours of the central nervous system (males and females)	–	1.2	–
Carcinoma of the thyroid	0.3		1.0

Histological sections were examined in every case where a classification was considered valuable, and when difficulties were encountered, several pathologists examined the sections.

A study such as this clearly has many pitfalls. Based as it is, entirely on pathological diagnosis in the laboratory, cases of clinical cancer in which no biopsy had been taken would be omitted from the study. Such examples include hepatocellular carcinoma where serological tests are eliminating the need for biopsy in a percentage of cases, and tumours of the lung which for various reasons are not all biopsied.

Results

Digestive System

Squamous Carcinoma of the Tongue

Tumours of the tongue are almost invariably squamous carcinomas showing varying degrees of differentiation. There is a marked male preponderance, 92% of cases being males. Seventy-five percent are over the age of 40 years. An occasional case occurring under the age of 30 is seen in very young children with xeroderma pigmentosum, in which the aetiological factors are clearly different from those operating in adults. Table 6.1 demonstrates the age specific incidence rates in males and females respectively. There is a comparatively high incidence in males whereas in females the incidence is extremely low. These figures are very similar to those of *Higginson* and *Oettle* (1960) who found that the incidence in Blacks in South Africa is probably less than in United States Whites.

Squamous Carcinoma of the Floor of the Mouth and Cheek

This tumour is also predominantly one of males over the age of 40 years. There were 83 males and 6 females. The tumour is comparatively infrequent with a considerably lower incidence than that seen in California Blacks or Whites. The tumour is rare in females (Table 6.1). These findings are not in accord with those of *Higginson* and *Oettle* (1960) who found that the incidence was similar to that in the United States Negro.

Salivary Glands

One hundred and forty-three tumours of salivary glands were found in the ten year survey. The sites of origin are shown in Table 6.2. Forty-nine percent of the tumours arose in the parotid compared with the 47% of *Higginson* and *Oettle* (1960). These findings confirm the observations of other workers that compared with White patients, Blacks are more frequently affected by tumours of salivary gland tissue other than the parotid (*Davies* et al. 1964). Twenty-four percent arose in the submandibular gland, a figure very similar to that reported by *Davies* et al. (1964) from Uganda, who found 52.7% arising in the parotid and 19.4% in the submandibular. The histological types of salivary gland tumours are shown in Table 6.3. There is a remarkable absence of adenolymphomas, not one tumour being found in the ten year survey. This is similar to the findings in Uganda (*Davies* et al. 1964). Ninety of the cases were females and 53 males.

There were 97 pleomorphic adenomas and their age distribution and site are shown in Table 6.4. Twenty-two percent of the tumours arose from minor salivary

Table 6.2. Distribution of all salivary gland tumours (benign and malignant)

Age in years	Parotid	Submandibular	Minor	Age unknown	Total
0– 9	1	2	1	0	4
10–19	6	2	3	1	12
20–29	13	8	4	0	25
30–39	12	7	6	2	27
40–49	14	6	9	1	30
50–59	9	5	6	0	20
60+	6	2	1	0	9
No age	9	3	2	2	16
Total	70	35	32	6	143

Table 6.3. Histological types of salivary gland tumours and sex distribution

	No of cases	% of total	Females	Males
Benign pleomorphic adenomas	97	67	63	34
Malignant pleomorphic adenomas	4	3	1	3
Adenoid cystic carcinoma	9	6.5	6	3
Mucoepidermoid tumours	18	12.6	11	7
Benign mucoepidermoid tumours	11	8	7	4
Malignant mucoepidermoid carcinoma	7	4.6	4	3
Pure adenocarcinoma (papillary and cystic)	4	3	0	4
Salivary duct carcinoma	1	0.7	1	0
Undifferentiated carcinoma	4	3	4	0
Acinic cell tumour	1	0.7	1	0
Benign oncocytic adenoma	1	0.7	1	0
Benign cystadenoma	1	0.7	1	0
Benign neurilemmoma	1	0.7	0	1
Benign myxoma	1	0.7	0	1
Inadequate for diagnosis	1	0.7	1	0
Total	143		90	53

glands which corresponds closely to the 25.6% in the Ugandan series (*Davies* et al. 1964). The number of palatal tumours is not high which is at variance with other series from Africa. Nine pleomorphic adenomas (4 males and 5 females) showed the presence of tyrosine crystals (*Nochomovitz* and *Kahn* 1974). Table 6.5 depicts the malignant tumours in this series which constituted 20% of the total. Table 6.1 demonstrates the age specific incidence of salivary gland tumours. There is a predominance of females and salivary gland tumours are slightly more frequent in Soweto Blacks than in California Blacks or Whites and occur with the same frequency as in England and Wales. *Higginson* and *Oettle* (1960) found that tumours of the salivary gland were not significantly more frequent among the Blacks of South Africa than in the U.S. population and *Davies* et al. (1964) found that the incidence of salivary gland tumours in Ugandan Africans was no higher than in non-African countries. *Higginson* and *Oettle* (1960) found 17% to be carcinomas as compared with the 20% in this series.

Squamous Carcinoma of the Oesophagus

Up to 25 years ago carcinoma of the oesophagus was comparatively rare in the Black population. At the South African Institute for Medical Research in Johannesburg from 1912 to 1927 no cases of oesophageal cancer were diagnosed in a Black patient, although over 200 primary hepatocellular carcinomas of the liver were encountered. In the 3 year survey of *Higginson* and *Oettle* (1960), 53 oesophageal cancer and 114 hepatocellular carcinomas were diagnosed. In recent years the ratio of oesophageal cancer to hepatocellular carcinoma has reversed and in 1960 the records of the histopathology laboratory at Baragwanath Hospital yielded 87 oesophageal carcinomas and 22 hepatocellular carcinomas (*Oettle* 1964).

Table 6.4. Pleomorphic adenomas of salivary glands

Age (years)	Parotid – 44		Submandibular – 27		Minor– 21 Palate – 11		Minor– 21 Others – 10		Unspecified – 5		
	M	F	M	F	M	F	M	F	M	F	Total
0– 9	0	0	1	0	0	0	1	0	0	0	2
10–19	1	2	1	1	2	0	1	0	0	0	8
20–29	3	7	4	3	1	1	0	0	0	0	19
30–39	2	6	1	4	0	2	1	1	0	2	19
40–49	2	5	1	3	0	2	1	2	0	1	17
50–59	2	4	2	3	1	0	2	0	0	0	14
60+	0	3	2	0	0	0	0	1	0	0	6
Unknown	1	6	0	1	1	1	0	0	0	2	12
Total	11	33	12	15	5	6	6	4	0	5	97

The high incidence of oesophageal cancer occurs in both rural and urban populations so that the carcinogenic stimulus is neither perculiarly urban nor perculiarly rural (*Oettle* 1963). The urban cases cannot be accounted for by recent migration from rural areas. In a Johannesburg survey the average length of urbanization of male patients with oesophageal cancer was 19.5 years compared with 16.9 years in controls with cancer of other parts of the body matched for age (*Oettle* 1963). *Schonland* and *Bradshaw* (1969) showed that oesophageal cancer is as frequent among Zulus of Natal as it is amongst the Xhosas, and that it is the commonest cancer among Natal Black males, comprising 18.3% of all male cancers. It is far less common among Natal Black females and comprises only 4.6% of all females cancers. In their series the incidence rose to peak at 45 to 64 years, and the commonest site was the thoracic oesophagus.

This series yielded 1331 cases of squamous carcinoma (1110 males and 221 females) and 11 cases of adenocarcinoma. The peak age incidence of squamous carcinoma is in the sixth decade but significant numbers are already present in the fourth decade and there are even a few cases in the third decade. Eighty one percent of cases occurred in subjects over the age of 40 years. The ratio of males to females is 5:1. Adenocarcinoma is rare. Table 6.1 shows the age specific incidence rates. The Soweto

Table 6.5. Malignant tumours of salivary glands

		F	M
Malignant pleomorphic adenoma	4	1	3
Malignant muco-epidermoid	7	4	3
Adenoid cystic carcinoma	9	6	3
Pure adenocarcinoma	4	0	4
Salivary duct carcinoma	1	1	0
Undifferentiated carcinoma	4	4	0
Total (20% of all cases)	29	16	13

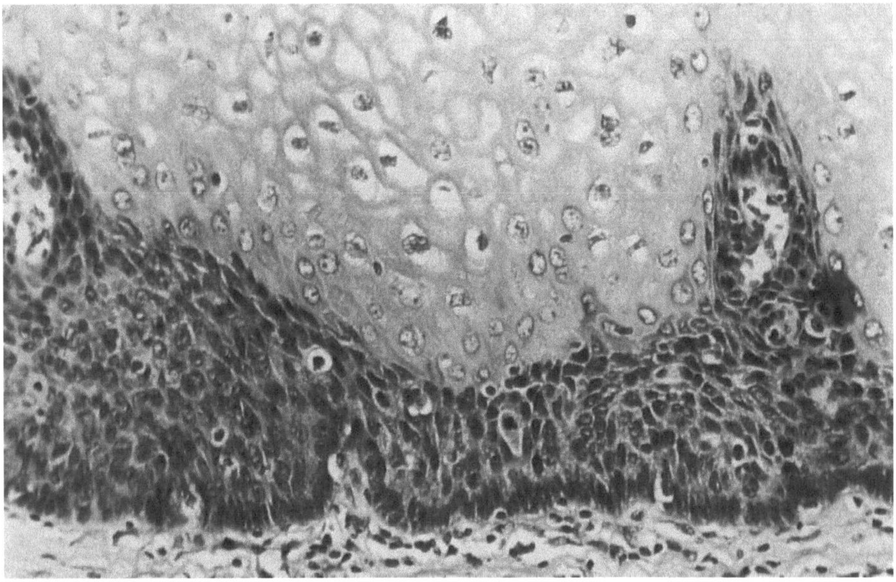

Fig. 6.1. High power view of basal cell atypia with loss of polarity and increased mitotic activity. The changes commence in the deeper layers of the squamous epithelium and sometimes infiltrative carcinoma has supervened before diffuse carcinoma in situ becomes manifest. H&E, ×280

Blacks show a strikingly high incidence in the younger are groups by comparison with other countries.

The records at the hospital do not permit an analysis of the site within the oesophagus of each carcinoma. Histologically, these tumours present the usual features of epidermoid carcinomas. A majority of the tumours produces significant quantities of keratin, but no significant correlation between keratinization and prognosis has even been shown. In some cases the infiltrating carcinoma is associated with carcinoma in situ in the overlying and adjacent squamous epithelium.

A common histological finding in the epithelium is that of increased activity and atypia of the basal cells with sprouts of squamous epithelium extending downwards into the subepithelial tissue, suggesting that the carcinoma starts in the deep layers of the squamous epithelium (Fig. 6.1). Squamous metaplasia, and occasionally carcinoma in situ may be seen in the underlying glands. Some tumours produce large quantities of keratin which provokes a foreign body giant cell reaction. This is seen particularly following radio-therapy. The tumour infiltrates throughout the thickness of the oesophagus and also insidiously beneath the overlying epithelium. Tumours in the region of the cardia may thus infiltrate beneath the mucosa of the stomach. "Swiss-roll" sections of the oesophagus reveal that the basal cell activity and dysplasia may be a field effect involving the entire length of the oesophagus and even the posterior one third of the tongue.

The aetiology of the high incidence of carcinoma of the oesophagus remains obscure. *Oettle* (1964) suggested a strong correlation with smoking, especially cigarettes, and a low one with drinking. The Blacks have consumed alcohol for generations yet the increase in oesophageal cancer is only recent. It may be of significance that in South Africa between 1941 and 1949, tin plating of kerosene containers was abandoned in favour of lead plating (*Oettle* 1964). There are a variety of oesophageal insults to which Black males are particularly prone and these include emetics, cigarettes and pipe smoking and concoction drinking (*McGlashan* et al. 1968). *McGlashan* and *Walters* (1969) suggested that nitrosamine contamination of alcoholic drinks could be a factor. *Burrell* et al. (1966) felt that molybdenum deficiency in the soil may lead to the formation of nitrosamines in the silage.

Recently *Ivankovic* et al. (1975) have suggested a possible pathogenetic pathway for the production of oesophageal cancer by nitrosamines. They have shown experimentally that carcinogenesis by ethyl nitrosourea (ENU) formed in vivo can be prevented by simultaneous administration of ascorbic acid. Ascorbic acid depletion associated with iron overload is common in this population. *Boyland* and *Walker* (1975) have suggested that there is an increased risk of nitrosamine formation in the stomach of smokers than in non smokers. The increased incidence of cancer in smokers could be due to increased formation of nitrosamines in the stomach. Recently it has been suggested that mouldy cereals may be a factor. Fusarium extracts may contain carcinogenic substances and ingestion of metabolites of this and other moulds may play a part in the causation of oesophageal cancer (The Lancet 1974; *Schoental* and *Joffe* 1974; *Crespi* et al. 1979; *Marsas* et al. 1979; *Mingxin* et al. 1979).

Stomach

Carcinoma of the stomach shows a marked male preponderance with 81 males out of 110 cases. The greatest incidence occurs over the age of 60 years. The survey also yielded four leiomyosarcomas and two lymphomas. Carcinomas are excessively rare up to the end of the fourth decade. Sixty of the carcinomas of the stomach were of the so-called diffuse or anaplastic type and 50 of the intestinal type. *Lauren* (1965) and *Munoz* et al. (1968) have demonstrated that the intestinal type predominates where the incidence of carcinoma is high, while the diffuse type is relatively more frequent where the incidence is low, the intestinal type being responsible for much of the difference between high and low risk areas. *Templeton* (1973) working in Uganda found a similar distribution of histological types with 88 of the intestinal type and 72 of the diffuse type. Table 6.1 demonstrates the age specific incidence rates for males and females. The incidence in this population is extremely low (*Higginson* and *Oettle* 1960). *Wynder* et al. (1963) claimed that gastric cancer appears more commonly in low socio-economic groups. *Higginson* (1968) stated that on the one hand it would seem that cancer of the stomach becomes less frequent where modern processing is in extensive use and on the other hand, cancer of the stomach is even more rare in countries eating a simple unprocessed diet as in Africa. The known precursor lesions of carcinoma of the stomach, such as intestinal metaplasia and chronic atrophic gastritis are also rare in this population.

Table 6.6. Carcinoma of the large bowel

Site	Males	Females	Total
Right colon	46	18	64
Left colon	19	18	37
Rectum	61	61	122
Total	126	97	223

Large Bowel

Tumours of the colon were reported to be rare among the South African Blacks in the period prior to 1953 (*Higginson* and *Oettle* 1960). With the process of urbanization and the introduction of a more Western type diet, this incidence would be expected to be on the increase. However, the survey at Baragwanath Hospital failed to reveal any demonstrable increase over a twenty year period. Two hundred and forty eight carcinomas were found, the average age being 51 years. The average age of the mucinous carcinomas was 42 years and thenon-mucinous 55 years. The peak age incidence was in the 50–60 year age group and the male-female ratio was 7:5. The anatomical distribution of the 223 cases in which it was known is shown in Table 6.6. Males predominated in tumours of the right colon by a ratio of 2.6:1, whereas the ratios in the left colon and rectum were 1:1. Tumours from different parts of the large bowel were histologically similar. Mucinous tumours comprised 20% of the total. Fifty percent of mucinous tumours occurred on the right side. Ten years of large bowel carcinoma were then examined in greater detail. The tumours were divided into rectal and colonic carcinomas. There were 32 rectal tumours in males, 35 rectal tumours in females, 40 tumours of colon in males and 18 in females. Table 6.1 shows the age specific incidence rates. The tumours occurred from the third decade onwards but were most frequent over the age of 40. The incidence of large bowel carcinoma in this population is one of the lowest in the world, and contrasts vividly with the rates in other racial groups in South Africa where the incidence amongst Whites is approximately 10 per 100,000. It has been suggested that large bowel cancer, diverticular disease and ulcerative colitis are all rare in communities which exist on a high residue diet, and common in every country where the low residue has been adopted. *Walker* (1971) has pointed out that the mean time of traversal of digested food in Africans is 2 to 3 times faster than in Caucasians. There is also a far greater frequency of motions in Blacks than in Caucasians and rural Africans have 2–3 motions daily in 30% of subjects compared with 1 to 2% in the case of Caucasians. Both *Walker* (1971) and *Burkitt* (1969) feel that the most important factor in the low incidence of colonic carcinoma in Blacks is the high dietary fibre content. *Bremner* and *Ackerman* (1970) reported that not only was large bowel cancer extremely rare, but intestinal polyps were also very infrequent. This is of importance in view of *Morson's* (1976) view that most intestinal cancers arise from benign polyps. *MacIllmurray* and *Langman* (1975) suggested that of the many factors studied only dietary constituents, particularly the proportion of animal proteins and fat, have been shown to correlate well with the geographical variations in the incidence of large bowel cancer.

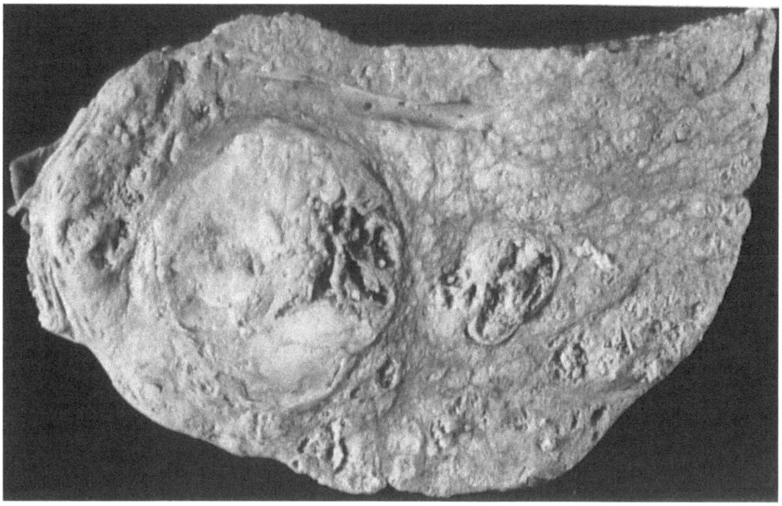

Fig. 6.2. Macroscopic appearance of hepatocellular carcinoma in a macronodular cirrhosis

The persistently low incidence in this Black population may be due to an absence of significant alteration in the dietary habits despite urbanization.

Hepatocellular Carcinoma

There were 281 cases – 238 males and 43 females – a male:female ratio of 5.5:1. The specimens examined included biopsies and autopsies. The cases were categorized according to age, sex and histological type, the presence or absence of cirrhosis, iron and bile.

The tumour is commonest over the age of 40 years although numbers of cases occurred in the third decade. In the majority of cases (75%) the growth presented the characteristic trabecular pattern with cylindrical cords and trabeculae of eosinophilic tumour cells resembling liver cells (Figs. 6.2–6.4). Six cases presented a clear cell structure (Fig. 6.5) and bile pigment was observed in only 4 cases. The carcinoma was associated with a macronodular cirrhosis in 115 cases (40%) and a micronodular cirrhosis in only 4 cases. Cirrhosis was absent in 18 cases and in 125 the material was insufficient for an assessment of the presence of cirrhosis. Dysplastic cells in the non-neoplastic liver were found in 43 cases (Fig. 6.6). Iron overload was present in very few cases confirming that beer consumption (from which the bulk of the iron is derived) plays no significant role in the aetiology of hepatocellular carcinoma. Malignant hepatoma is still an extremely common tumour in Blacks, although recent studies show that there has been a drop in the incidence in Shangaan miners from Mozambique (*Bradshaw* and *Harington* 1976).

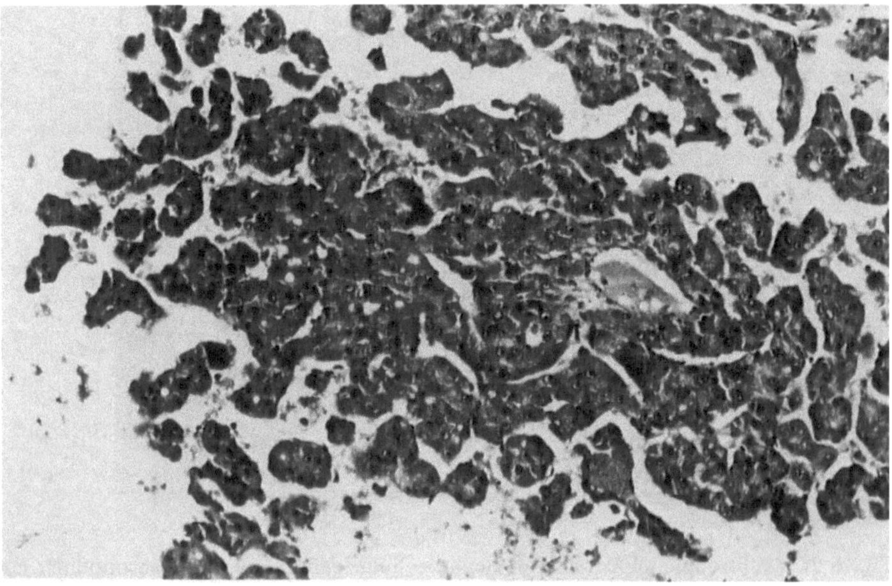

Fig. 6.3. Hepatocellular carcinoma showing a trabecular pattern. H&E, × 175

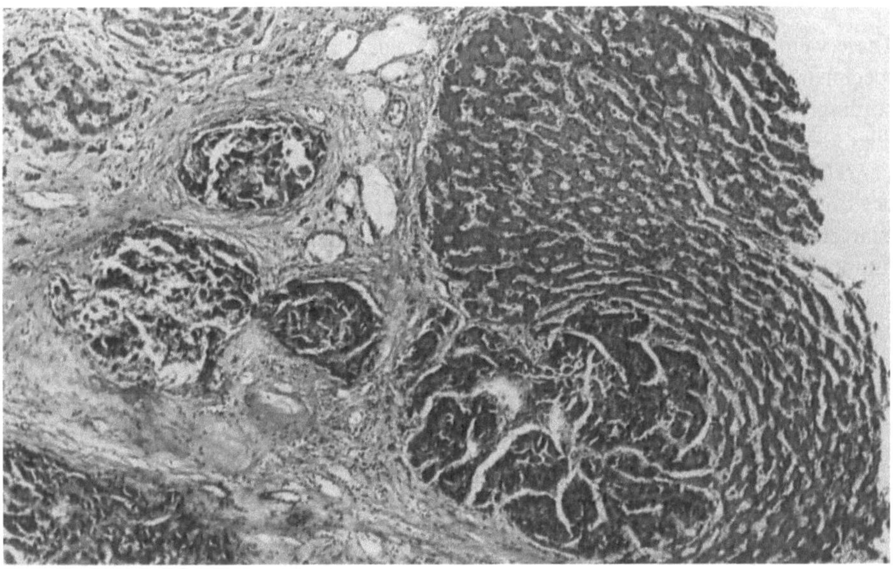

Fig. 6.4. Hepatocellular carcinoma in a cirrhotic liver. The tumour mimics the structure of normal liver. H&E, × 70

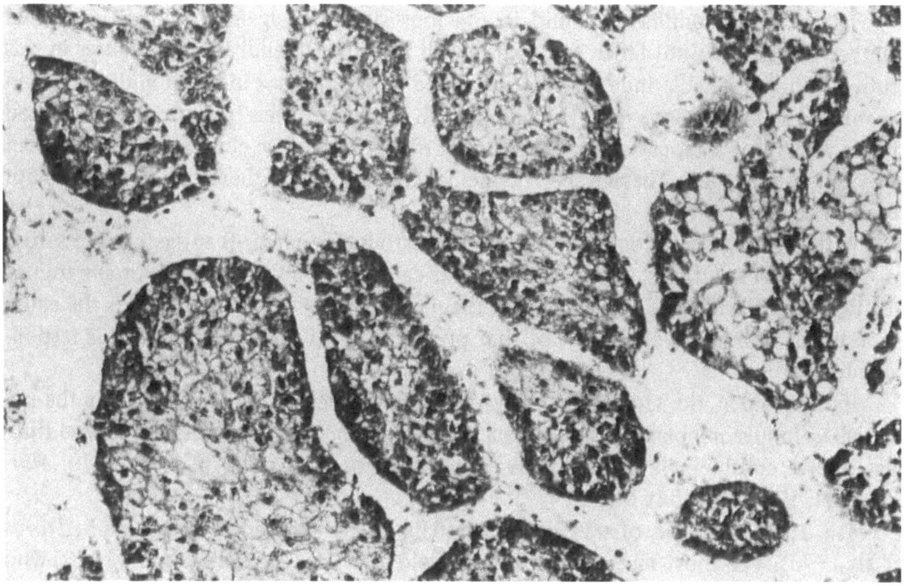

Fig. 6.5. Hepatocellular carcinoma with many clear cells. H&E, × 175

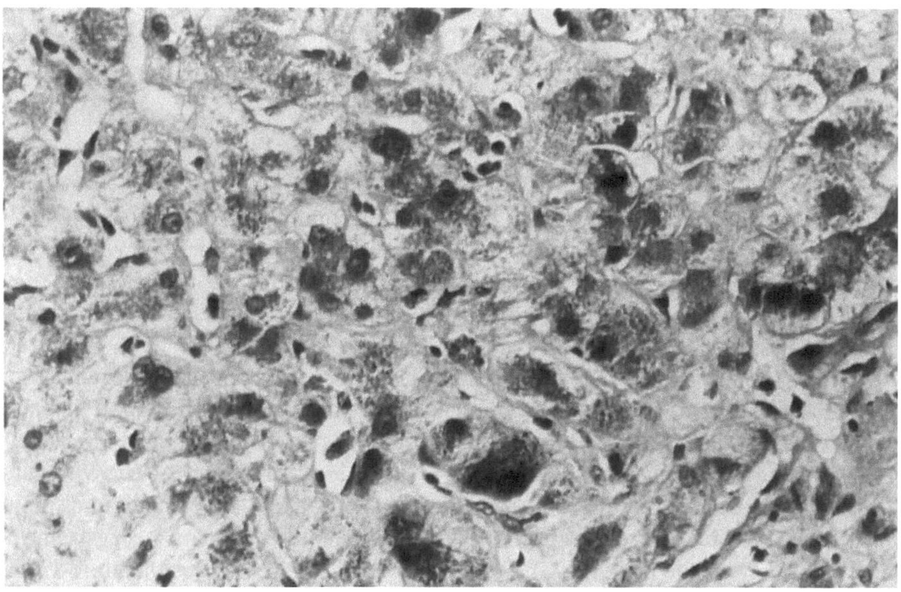

Fig. 6.6. Dysplastic cells in vicinity of hepatocellular carcinoma. H&E, × 410

The male predominance found in previous studies is again striking. The annual number of cases has not fallen at Baragwanath Hospital. In addition, the figures in this study are not a reliable index of the incidence of the tumour in this population, as in recent years the extensive use of the alpha-feto protein test has in many cases obviated the necessity for a biopsy. The true number of cases could be considerably more than depicted in this study. The age specific incidence rates should therefore be viewed with reserve (Table 6.1).

With regard to aetiology, *Kew* et al. (1974) found hepatitis B antigen in the serum of 40% of Black patients with hepatocellular carcinoma, but in only 7% of apparently healthy rural Blacks, and suggested that the persistence of hepatitis B virus is the cause or result of primary liver cancer, or that possibly some immunologic defect is responsible for both.

If the former, the virus must be directly oncogenic, in addition to having the potential to induce neoplasia indirectly via chronic parenchymal liver disease. These findings receive considerable support from other parts of Africa (*Vogel* et al. 1970; *Morrow* et al. 1971; *Anthony* et al. 1972).

The aflatoxin thesis of aetiology has equally many adherents (*Oettle* 1965; *Torres* et al. 1970). The most recent work in this field is by *Van Resnburg* et al. (1975) who examined the relationship between the level of aflatoxin intake and the primary liver cancer rate. Working in the Imhambane district of Mozambique, the area with the highest known liver cancer incidence in the world, they found that the diet contains the highest aflatoxin intake.

Most workers agree that the aetiology of hepatocellular carcinoma is multifactorial and is probably a combination of mycotoxins and hepatitis B virus.

Respiratory System

Carcinoma of the Nasal Sinuses

There were 60 cases, 48 males and 12 females. The tumours were all squamous carcinomas and occurred predominantly over the age of 40 years. Twenty nine arose from the maxillary antrum, 5 from the ethmoid sinus, one from the frontal sinus, three from the post nasal space, and in 22 the site of origin was not stated in the available clinical notes.

It has been suggested that the relatively high frequency in males is dependent on the inhalation of snuff to which additional ingredients, notably burnt vegetable matter, are usually added (*Keen* et al. 1955). From this snuff known carcinogens have been isolated (*Higginson* and *Oettle* 1960). However, in the series of *Higginson* and *Oettle* (1960) nearly half the cases denied using snuffs, and other carcinogenic stimuli may be involved. There were also 25 cases of squamous carcinoma arising from the nose and 48 from the pharynx. The total number of antral cases was therefore 133 of which 30 were females. The age specific incidence rates for males and females are seen in Table 6.1.

Larynx

Higginson and *Oettle* (1960) stated that this cancer is significantly less common in Johannesburg Blacks than United States Whites and Negroes. This survey indicates that the tumour is not rare, 186 cases being found (175 males and 11 females). All the tumours were squamous carcinomas and the majority were found in males over the age of 40 years. In males the tumour is only slightly less frequent than in Denmark, but the incidence is less than that of Californian Blacks and Californian Whites. The tumour is rare in females.

Carcinoma Bronchus

There were 193 cases of bronchial carcinoma of which 170 were males and 23 females. Nearly half the tumours were squamous carcinomas. Age specific incidence rates for bronchogenic carcinoma were not computed for this series as the number is not a true reflection of the clinical incidence of the disease. For various reasons a significant percentage of bronchogenic carcinomas were not biopsied and treatment was not infrequently instituted on the basis of the clinical and radiological findings alone. In Natal lung cancer is one of the commonest tumours in Black males, in some areas comprising 20% of all male malignancies (*Schonland* and *Bradshaw* 1969). The Durban Black male has an incidence of lung cancer approaching the level measured in England and the tumour is becoming as great a problem as oesophageal cancer.

A prospective combined cytological, histopathological, clinical and radiological study at this hospital has yielded approximately 100 cases in one year. The majority of these were males. These preliminary figures indicate a combined male – female incidence very close to that of carcinoma of the oesophagus.

Carcinoma of the Breast

There is a low relative frequency of breast cancer in the Blacks of Southern Africa (*Higginson* and *Oettle* 1960). *Oettle* (1964) claimed that breast cancer was less than one quarter of that in U.S. Whites, and the incidence in males is not elevated despite the frequency of gynecomastia. *Pearson* (1963) from Nigeria suggested that the tumours amongst Nigerian women are more highly malignant than among Caucasians, which would account for the observation that the growths are generally more advanced than usual by the time the patients reach hospital. *Burkitt* (1971) has stated that both malignant and benign lesions of the breast are much less common in under developed countries where women not only have constantly recurring pregnancies, but where babies are breast fed for long periods. The close correlation between the incidence of breast and colon cancer and a high standard of living has led many people to suggest that dietary practice may be involved (*Hill* et al. 1971; *Doll* 1975).

This study yielded 357 cases of malignant tumours of the breast. There were 14 males, 3.9% of the total, which is no higher than in the equivalent Caucasian population. There were thus 343 breast malignancies in females of which 3 were sarcomas – a liposarcoma, a carcinosarcoma and an angiosarcoma – and 340 were carcinomas, an incidence rate of 6 per 100.000 (Table 6.1). No significant change in the number of cases diagnosed annually was seen over the ten years.

The carcinomas were graded according to the WHO method and no significant difference was found in the nuclear grading between Soweto Blacks and those from Japan or the United States (*Chabon* et al. 1974). These findings indicate that breast carcinoma in Blacks is not more aggressive as compared with other population groups, and the poor therapeutic results are probably due to patients presenting themselves late for treatment rather than African breast cancer having a heightened degree of malignancy (*Davies* 1970). The age distribution was similar to that in Caucasians.

Different histological types were compared with the series by *Fisher* et al. (1975) from the United States. The same histological classification was employed and the distribution in the two series was very similar. *Fisher* et al. (1975) had a higher percentage of infiltrating duct with combinations, which probably reflects the greater number of histological sections examined. Medullary carcinoma is rarer in Blacks and adenocystic carcinoma was not seen. These findings indicate that although breast carcinoma in the Black female is considerably less frequent than in the equivalent Caucasian population, the histological types and grading do not vary significantly from other population groups.

Female Genital Tract

Cervix Uteri

Carcinoma of the cervix is the commonest malignant tumour in Black females, in whom it accounts for 41.7% of all cancers (*Higginson* and *Oettle* 1960). This is in striking contrast to the low frequency of carcinoma of the body of the uterus. Bilharzia is not a promoting factor and circumcision of male partners may be an effective preventative factor for cervix cancer, although the rate of cancer of the cervix in Moslems is unexpectedly high in view of the fact that Moslems practise circumcision (*Schonland* and *Bradshaw* 1968).

TeGroen and *Rose* (1974) found that among the Black population of the Eastern Cape Province where circumcision is practised widely, the rate of carcinoma of the cervix is extremely high, suggesting that circumcision in male partners does not offer any protection against cervical cancer. *Freedman* et al. (1974) found an association between carcinoma of the cervix and HSVII infection among Black patients, but could find no relationship between carcinoma of the cervix and bilharzia. Their results were inconclusive in relation to the role of trichomonas. Age at first coitus and at first marriage, and promiscuity were very strongly associated with the development of the disease, and socio-economic status, genital hygiene and venereal disease also played a major part. Circumcision of the male partner is, at best weakly associated with the development of the disease.

Recently *Harington* (1975) isolated a group of potent carcinogens – nitrosamines – in infected discharges of samples taken from the vaginal vault of patients attending a gynaecologic clinic. No significance can as yet be attached to the amount of nitros-

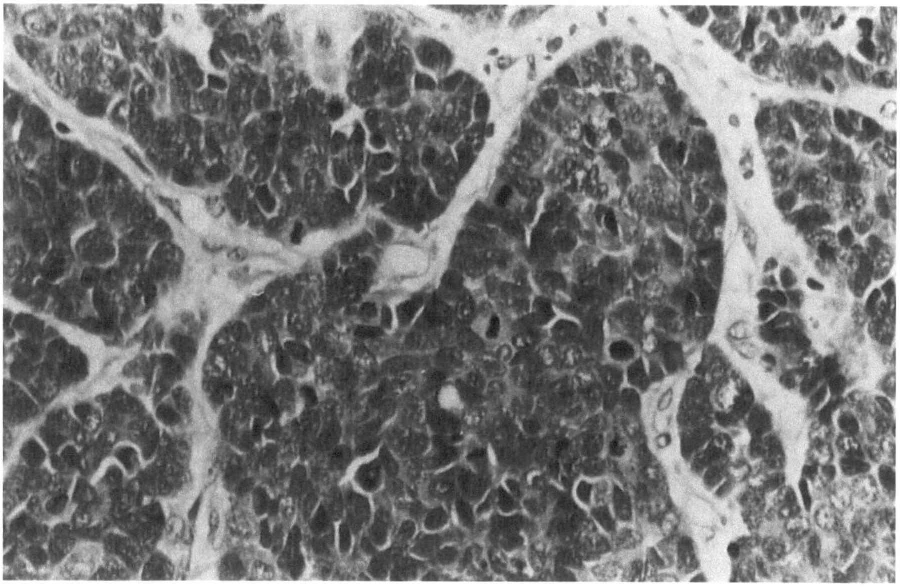

Fig. 6.7. High power view of large cell non keratinizing squamous carcinoma. The islands of tumour cells have blunt edges and show comparatively little pleomorphism although mitoses are frequent in this section. H&E, ×410

amines detected nor can any conclusions be drawn as to whether the findings implicate trichomonas vaginalis in the production of nitrosamines.

In the case of carcinoma of the cervix, only five years of material were examined and these yielded 550 cases of invasive squamous carcinoma. The tumour is not infrequently seen in the third decade, although the peak incidence is in the fifth decade (Table 6.1). Of the 550 cases, 419 (76%) were of the large cell non keratinizing type and 123 (22%) of the keratinizing type (Figs. 6.7, 6.8). There were 8 cases of small cell carcinoma.

The subdivision of squamous carcinoma of the cervix into large cell non-keratinizing, keratinizing and small cell varieties is of doubtful value (*Ng* and *Atkins* 1973; *Reagan* 1974). Recent studies (*Gunderson* et al. 1974; *de Moor* and *Berry* 1976) relate survival in carcinoma of the cervix to clinical stage and efficacy of treatment, rather than to histological pattern. Great difficulty was also experienced in delineating the very early stages of micro-invasive squamous carcinoma of the cervix. When micro-invasive carcinoma was defined in terms of depth of infiltration and was manifest by clear cut infiltrative islands of squamous carcinoma, no difficulty was experienced (Fig. 6.9) but when the carcinoma was still apparently confined to the in situ position but showed early cytological evidence of micro-invasion (*Roche* and *Norris* 1975; *Rubio* et al. 1974) difficulty was experienced in definitely diagnosing this condition. In many instances the maturation of the epithelial cells with the cytoplasmic eosinophilia and the development of nucleoli which have been described in micro invasive carcinoma, could be found in foci of undoubted in situ carcinoma (Fig. 6.10). The

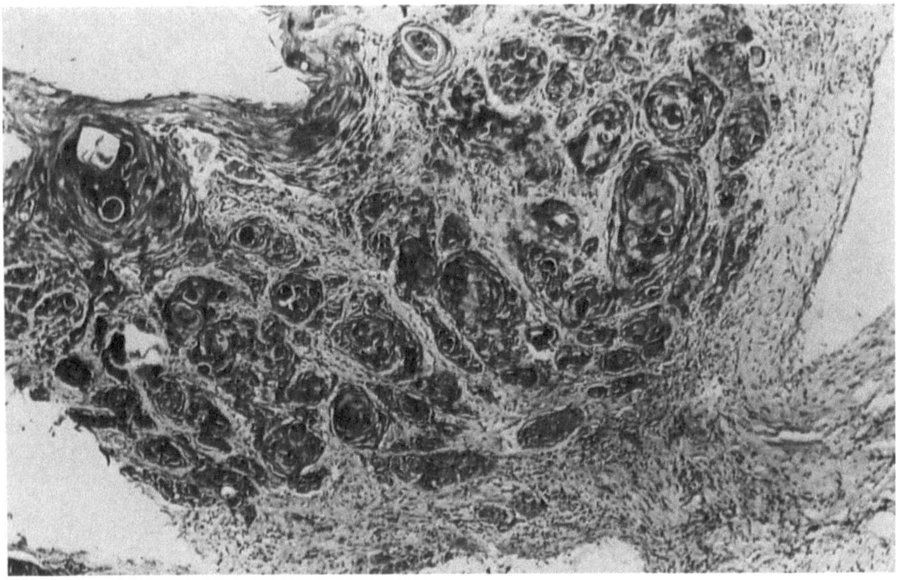

Fig. 6.8. Keratinizing squamous carcinoma of the cervix with numerous epithelial pearls. H&E, ×70

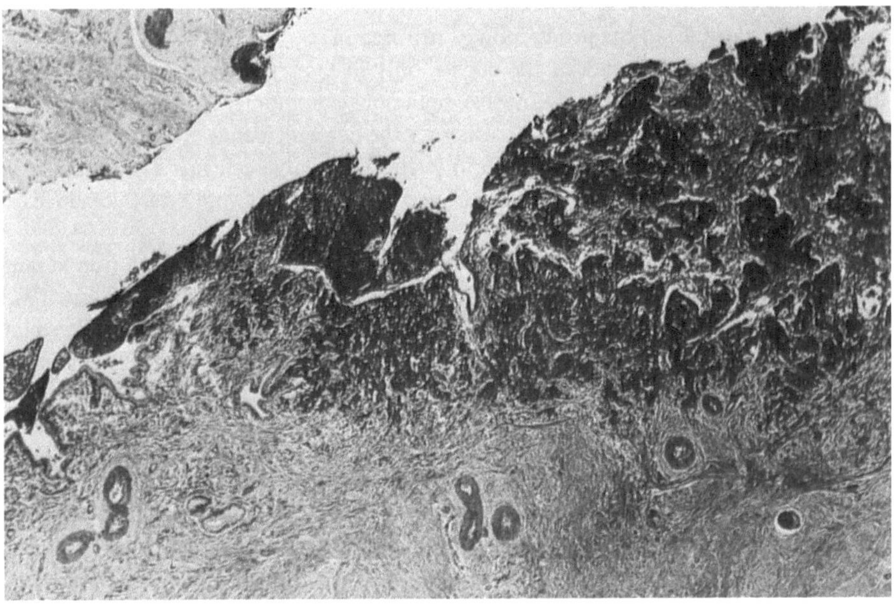

Fig. 6.9. Micro-invasive squamous carcinoma extending into the underlying stroma for a distance of about 2 mm. Clear cut infiltrating islands of invasive carcinoma are present. H&E, ×28

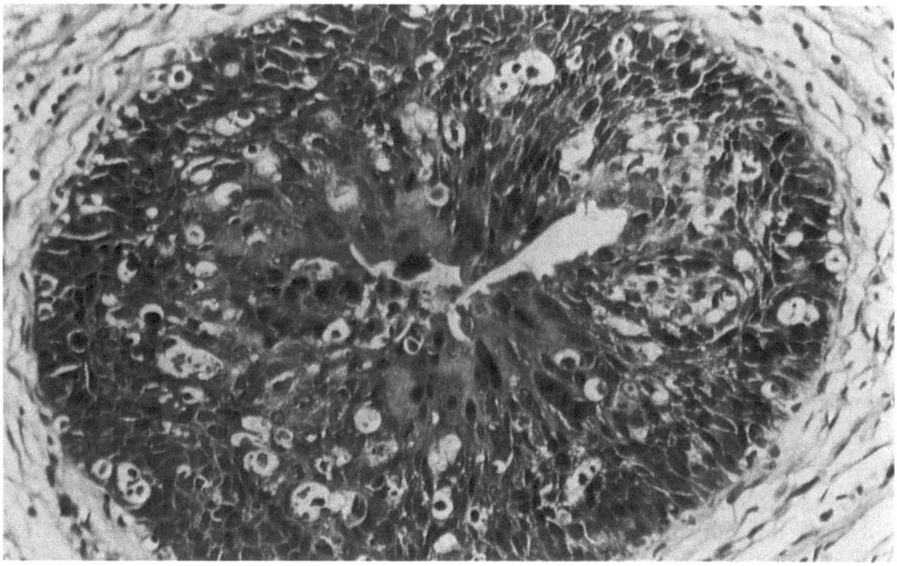

Fig. 6.10. Focus of carcinoma in situ in which nevertheless some of the epithelial cells show maturation to a more squamoid pattern with cytoplasmic eosinophilia and the development of nucleoli. H&E, × 270

premise that one is able to diagnose micro invasion on the basis of early cytological abnormalities seems to be very tenuous.

Adenocarcinoma of the cervix is a rare tumour only 37 cases being found in the five years. It usually occurs in women over the age 30 years.

There were 342 cases of squamous carcinoma in situ during the same five year period. The peak incidence of carcinoma in situ is a decade lower than that for invasive carcinoma.

Corpus Uteri

Higginson and *Oettle* (1960) commented on the extremely low frequency of carcinoma of the corpus uteri in Blacks, their survey yielding only one diagnosed case. This series comprised 71 cases, the ratio of invasive squamous carcinoma of the cervix to endometrial carcinoma being 15:1. This is a tumour of elderly women, 60 of the cases (84%) occurring over the age of 50 years. Table 6.1 demonstrates the age specific incidence rates. The rate for California Whites is 29 times higher than that for Soweto Blacks.

Mixed Mesodermal Tumours of the Uterus

The incidence of these tumours is not different from other populations although the small numbers makes a statistical analysis impossible. There were 8 cases and the majority of the tumours occurred in women over the age of 50 years.

Chorionepithelioma

Higginson and *Oettle* (1960) suggested that the incidence of chorionepithelioma was higher than that in Europeans and Americans. *Oettle* (1964) found the rate to be 1 per 7440 births, as compared with Western groups of 1 in 40,000–160,000. *Junaid* et al. (1974) claimed that chorioncarcinoma is the third most common malignant tumour in Nigerian females, and that it is more frequent than malignant ovarian neoplasms but less frequent than cervical and breast cancer. This series yielded 11 cases. Table 6.1 demonstrates the age specific incidence rate, which is much the same as California Whites and lower than California Blacks. These findings fail to demonstrate a high incidence of chorionepthelioma. The figures are in line with the rest of the world where the incidence of hydatidiform mole and chorionepithelioma run parallel (*Park* 1971). The incidence of hydatidiform mole in this population is no higher than in White subjects.

Ovary

Higginson and *Oettle* (1960) stated that ovarian tumours were much less frequent than would have been expected from a population in the United States or Denmark. *Grech* and *Lewis* (1967) reporting from Uganda found a low rate of serous and pseudomucinous cystadenomas and cystadenocarcinomas, with a high rate of malignant teratomas, granulosa cell tumours, dysgerminomas and Brenner tumours. *Bhoola* and *Bhamjee* (1976) from Durban compared ovarian tumours in Black and Indian patients and found a disparity in the incidence of cystomas and teratomas in the two groups, cystomas comprising 29% of all ovarian tumours in Blacks compared with 67% in Indians.

The Indian distribution was similar to that in American and European groups. Cystomas comprise 60% of all ovarian tumours in Americans and White South Africans. *Charlewood* and *Frylinck* (1951) found that teratomas, taken as a percentage of all ovarian tumours, constitute 24.5% in Whites and 45.5% in Blacks.

Five years of ovarian tumours were examined. There were 172 cases covering the period 1971–1975 of which ten were metastatic (Table 6.7). Nearly 60% of the primary tumours were of germ cell origin and more than half of the primary ovarian tumours were benign cystic teratomas. A striking feature was the small number of mucinous and serous papillary tumours. The overall age specific incidence rates are low suggesting that the high germ cell percentage is not absolute but due to the low number of cystomas.

Table 6.7. Tumours of the ovary

Year	Total	Benign cystic teratoma	Brenner tumour	Dysgermi-noma	Fibro thecoma	Fibro adenosis	Granulosa cell	Mesothelioma Malignant	Mesothelioma Benign	Inclu cyst	Mucinous Malignant	Mucinous Benign	Papillary serous
1971	31	14	4	1	1	1	0	3	3	2	0	0	1
1972	31	19	3	0	3	1	1	3	0	0	0	0	0
1973	35	18	9	0	1	0	1	3	0	0	1	0	1
1974	33	14	1	1	4	0	1	5	0	0	0	2	1
1975	42	19	1	2	6	0	0	5	1	4	0	2	0
	162	84	18	4	14	2	3	19	4	6	1	4	3
	10 Metastatic												

Male Genital System

Prostate

Higginson and *Oettle* (1960) found prostatic cancers to comprise 4.1% of all male cancers, a number similar to that expected at Danish rates but much lower than in United States White or Negroes. *Oettle* (1964) reported that in the Johannesburg Black the incidence of cancer of the prostate is about one fifth that of U.S. Non-Whites. *Wainwright* and *Roach* (1957) also reported a low incidence of prostatic carcinoma in the Natal African. Not everyone agrees with these findings (*Movsas* 1966).

This study yielded 246 cases of prostatic carcinoma, the histological features of which were essentially similar to those observed in other populations. There was one adenosquamous carcinoma, one mixed adenotransitional cell carcinoma, one squamous carcinoma and two endometriod carcinomas. The age specific incidence rates are seen in Table 6.1. The incidence is approximately one tenth of that in California Blacks. These figures are at variance with the views of *Higginson* and *Oettle* (1960) that the incidence is similar to that of Denmark. This study shows that the incidence in Blacks is not much lower than in Danes up to the seventh decade after which there is a marked disparity. This is not solely due to the smaller number of elderly Blacks.

In the years following this survey there has been a marked increase in the incidence of prostatic carcinoma, the number of cases almost doubling compared with the previous ten years. The cause of this is uncertain and no specific dietary or other environmental factor can be incriminated.

Testis

The incidence of this malignancy in the South African Black is extremely low (*Higginson* and *Oettle* 1960). Cancer of the testis, unlike most other genital tumours is rarer in United States Negro males than in the United States Whites (*Dixon* and *Moore* 1953). There were 8 malignant tumours in this study and one benign. The malignant tumours consisted of five seminomas, two teratomas and one embryonal carcinoma. Table 6.1. shows the age specific incidence which suggests that carcinoma of the testis in Blacks is independent of the environment, since Blacks living under quite different conditions all show a low incidence.

Penis

Approximately 42% of Black males in Soweto are circumcised and penile cancer accounts for 1.4% of all cancers. In Kenya where most of the male population is circumcised, penile cancer accounts for 1.9% of all male cancers (*Oettle* 1964). In Uganda where less than 10% of males are circumcised penile cancer accounts for 7.2% of all male cancers (*Dodge* 1965). The standardised incidence rate in Uganda is more than ten times that for Norway. The role of circumcision in the genesis of penile cancer in Africans in unequivocal (*Dodge* 1965).

In Kenya two tribes account for 15.8% of the population, but account for 77.8% of the cases of carcinoma of the penis, and these two tribes are the only two that do not observe the custom of circumcision. *Higginson* and *Oettle* (1960) felt that late circumcision has only a slight protective effect and a high percentage of Blacks who do undergo circumcision only do so at puberty or later. Circumcision forms part of the initiation ceremony which takes place during or after puberty and can therefore be expected to have less effect than circumcision in infancy. There were 61 cases in this study and the tumour occurs most frequently over the age of 40. All the tumours were squamous carcinomas. Table 6.1 shows the age specific incidence rates. The incidence is low, approximately one fortieth the rate for California Blacks. The rarity of carcinoma of the penis contrasts strikingly with the high incidence of carcinoma of the cervix.

Urinary System

Kidney

The incidence of renal cancer in South African Blacks is very low, the survey of *Higginson* and *Oettle* (1960) yielding only 5 cases as against the 24 expected in the U.S.A. However, nephroblastoma is as common as in the Western world. *Uys* (1956) found three renal carcinomas and two nephroblastomas in a series of 3707 consecutive autopsies. The usual ratio in Western countries of adenocarcinoma to nephroblastoma is 8:1. This relative frequency of nephroblastoma or infrequency of adenocarcinoma is seen in many parts of Africa (*Linsell* and *Martyn* 1962; *Davey* 1964; *Davies* et al. 1965).

There were 25 cases of renal cell carcinoma. No sex predilection was noted. There were 31 nephroblastomas, 3.1 cases per annum. No sex predilection was noted. The incidence of nephroblastoma does not differ from that in other populations. It is however higher than would be expected from the population of Soweto alone, but in the case of nephroblastomas it seems likely that some patients come from more remote areas. It has been suggested that 200,000–250,000 children under the age of 14 years yield one nephroblastoma annually regardless of the origin of the population (The Lancet 1973). If all the cases observed at Baragwanath Hospital were derived from Soweto, this would imply that the population of Soweto is not far short of 2 million. This is highly unlikely, and one must conclude that a significant number of the nephroblastomas originate from more remote areas. As in other populations studies, nearly all the tumours occurred in children under the age of six years. Table 6.1 depicts the average annual incidence per 100,000 of all malignant tumours of the kidney, i.e. renal cell carcinomas and nephroblastomas. The incidence is low, being approximately one sixth of California Blacks. This low incidence is clearly due to the very small number of renal cell carcinomas. As California Blacks develop significant numbers of renal cell carcinomas, it seems that some environmental factor must play a role in the aetiology of this tumour.

Bladder

In Uganda *Dodge* (1962) found no convincing evidence of a direct association between bladder cancer and bilharzia, although squamous carcinomas formed 34% of the proven carcinomas in his series. *Prates* and *Gillman* (1959) suggested that there is a predisposition in the urinary bladder of Black men to undergo squamous metaplasia whether bilharzia is present or not. *Hinder* and *Schmaman* (1969), writing from Baragwanath Hospital, found that the similarity in the incidence of bilharzial ova in the male population at risk (15.8%) and in those with transitional carcinoma of the bladder (18.6%) suggested that bilharzia plays no part in the genesis of this form of cancer. However, the incidence of bilharzia with squamous carcinoma (68.2%) confirmed the long held concept that bilharzia contributes to the development of squamous carcinoma. Bilharzial ova have been found to contain beta-glucoronidase which depolymerizes polysaccharides and might act on various precarcinogens found in the urine (*Fripp* 1965). *Higginson* and *Oettle* (1960) found 16 of their 23 bladder carcinomas to be of the squamous type. Transitional cell carcinomas were less frequent and transitional cell tumours in general were rare in urologic practice among the Blacks. *Schonland* and *Bradshaw* (1968) reported that bladder cancers in Africans and Indians are not common despite an endemic bilharzial infestation of about 30%.

There were 36 cases of transitional cell tumour of the bladder of which 28 were males. Only two of the 36 had associated bilharziasis. There were 38 cases of squamous carcinoma of the bladder, 30 males, and 21 showed bilharzial infestation. Table 6.1 shows the average annual incidence of combined transitional cell and squamous carcinomas. The combined incidence of transitional and squamous carcinomas is low despite the frequency of bilharzia. It is pertinent to add that the survey yielded only 2 cases of transitional cell tumours of the renal pelvis.

Skin

Whites have higher rates of skin cancer than the pigmented races particularly squamous cell carcinoma, basal cell carcinoma and melanoma, although adnexal tumours show no obvious racial differences (*Oettle* 1963). The higher rates observed in exposed areas of Whites and albino Blacks are mainly attributable to sunlight, as is indicated by the degree of actinic degeneration of the dermis. Keratoacanthoma and basal cell carcinoma are very rare in deeply pigmented races and there is a very low frequency of intradermal or junctional naevi in the Blacks of South Africa. Most squamous carcinomas develop from antecedent lesions such as tropical phagedenic ulceration, burns, scars, sinuses and fistulae. This survey yielded 101 cases of squamous carcinoma of the skin (59 males and 42 females). Seven of the subjects were albinos. Tumours occurred at virtually any age although they were commoner over the age of 40. The majority occurred in the head, neck and lower limbs. The clinical records could not supply an assessment of the number of cases that arose in burn sites. It is however, generally accepted that a high percentage of squamous carcinomas of the skin in Blacks arises in old scars commonly the result of burns (*Rippey* and *Schmaman* 1972).

Basal Cell Carcinoma

Basal cell carcinoma is extremely rare in Blacks, only 9 cases being found, 5 males and 4 females. One of the cases was a child of six years with xeroderma pigmentosum. Three of the subjects were albinos.

Malignant Melanoma

Rippey and *Schmaman* (1972) have accentuated the observation of earlier writers that malignant melanoma is predominantly a tumour of the sole of the foot in Blacks. They found that 80% occurred on the lower extremity, 13.6% on the head and neck and 1% on the abdominal wall. *Higginson* and *Oettle* (1960) showed that malignant melanoma was less frequent in the urban African who was more likely to wear shoes than in the rural African, and they thus invoked a traumatic aetiology. From Uganda, *Kariyabwire* (1968) reported that the commonest site of malignant melanoma was the sole of the foot where 64% of the cases occurred. This is however an area with little pigmentation. The presence of the majority of the tumours on the sole of the foot has led to a suggestion that trauma might be an important factor, although *Davies* et al. (1968) doubt whether urbanization and shoe-wearing in Johannesburg has altered the rate of melanoma. In the series of *Giraud* et al. (1975) from Johannesburg, 80.4% occurred in the lower extremity, predominantly the foot. In Queensland, Australia, only 2.4% occurred on the foot (*Beardmore* 1972).

This series yielded 83 cases with a high percentage occurring on the lower limb, 62 being described as arising from the foot, and in the majority this indicated the sole of the foot; eight were described as arising from the leg, the precise anatomical area not being stated, but the sole of the foot was probably the site in the majority. In 6 cases, the site of origin of the tumour was not stated in the protocols and it can be assumed that the sole of the foot was probably the most frequent. Of the remaining cases, only 5 arose from the upper extremity, 3 from the hand and 2 from the fingers; one arose from the lip and one from the nose. There is no sex predilection. Table 6.1 shows the age specific incidence rates. The frequency in males is considerably lower than in California Whites but is not dissimilar to California Blacks. If malignant melanoma could be eliminated from the feet of Blacks, the incidence would be extremely low.

Kaposi's Haemangiosarcoma

Kaposi's sarcoma is common amongst Negroid races of Africa (*Oettle* 1964). The increased susceptibility cannot be regarded as primarily genetic in view of the relative insusceptibility of American Negroes. The site and sex distribution suggest that the predominant factors are environmental. The incidence in Blacks of the Transvaal is about ten times that of Whites (*Oettle* 1962). *Oettle* (1962) claimed that Kaposi's sarcoma is encountered with approximately the same frequency as malignant melanoma and squamous carcinoma, and that it formed the commonest malignant tumour of

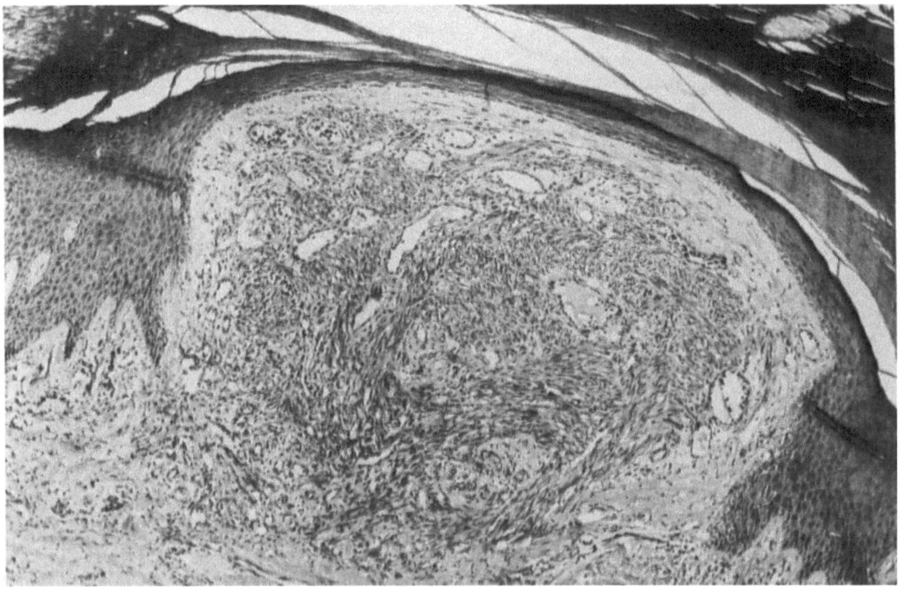

Fig. 6.11. Skin nodule in Kaposi's haemangiosarcoma showing numerous capillaries surrounded by interlacing whorls of fibroblastic like tissue. H&E, ×70

upper and lower limbs. *Davies* (1962) has stressed the male predominance of the disease. The tumour does not seem to occur in the albino or in xeroderma pigmentosum. More than 90% of cases occur in males, and it usually presents with vascular skin nodules of variable size, most marked in a peripheral distribution on the limbs.

This survey yielded 36 cases (32 males) making the tumour much less frequent than malignant melanoma or squamous carcinoma. Few cases occurred in the young, the majority being over the age of 40. The generalized visceral disease is infrequent in Blacks in Johannesburg and the mojority have lesions confined to the skin and subcutaneous tissue (Fig. 6.11). The incidence of this tumour has fallen considerably.

Central Nervous System

Proctor (1955) has drawn attention to the relative rarity of brain tumours among Blacks which appear with one fifth the frequency of Whites. *Higginson* and *Oettle* (1960) also found the number of brain tumours in Blacks significantly less than in United States Whites or Negroes. There is a higher proportion of meningiomas in Blacks than Whites (*Proctor* 1975; *Oettle* 1964). *Louis* and *Keet* (1964) found that expressed as numbers per million of each population group, there were 118 gliomas per million in the White population of South Africa, 19.2 per million in the Coloured population, and 4.3 in the Black population. Meningiomas occurred with approximately equal frequency in Whites (36 per million), and Coloureds (30 per million), while the figure is low for Blacks (2.6 per million). *Froman* and *Lipschitz* (1970) investigated the incidence of primary nervous system tumours over a twenty year period (1949–1968) at Baragwanath Hospital and reported a marked dearth of central nervous system tumours when comparisons were drawn with Caucasian populations.

This survey yielded 120 cases. The figure includes biopsies, autopsies and those clinically diagnosed but not biopsied. The latter category comprised only four cases in 1975, diagnosed on clinical grounds. No sex predilection was noted.

Fifty-four of the 120 cases were of the glioma series and 56 meningiomas, a meningioma–glioma ratio of 1:1. The pattern in Caucasian populations is generally a meningioma–glioma ratio of 1:2. *Froman* and *Lipschitz* (1970) in their series of 213 Black patients reported a meningioma–glioma ratio of 2:1. There were 36 astrocytomas, 8 ependymomas, 6 medulloblastomas, 4 oligodendrogliomas, 56 meningiomas, 3 craniopharyngiomas, 3 haemangiomas, 1 germinoma and 3 acoustic neuromas. The incidence is low, being less than one third that of California Blacks but is however, three times that of the Nigerians. An analysis of the age distribution shows two peaks, the first in the 0–9 year age group and the 2nd in the 40–49 year age group, similar to those cited in standard texts. Age specific incidence rates can be seen in Table 6.1.

Endocrine System

Thyrotoxicosis is very rare in Blacks, as is myxoedema, gigantism, acromegaly, pituitary dwarfism, adrenal virilism, Addison's disease, and all the classic endocrine disorders of Europe (*Davies* 1957). Although tuberculosis is frequent in Blacks, often fatal and disseminated, the adrenals are comparatively rarely affected, and in addition, cancer metastases in Blacks rarely involve the adrenal (*Davies* 1957). Functioning tumours of the endocrine glands are rare. *Wright* (1967) also commented on the rarity of thyrotoxicosis in the African and on the absence of lymphoid hyperplasia and focal thyroiditis, findings which are common in thyroid glands of White patients with thyrotoxicosis. Thyroid carcinoma among the Blacks of South Africa is rarer than in Caucasian populations, and the distribution is different with a preponderance of follicular tumours (*Decker* 1974). This survey yielded 68 cases of thyroid carcinoma. Table 6.1 demonstrates the average annual incidence per 100,000 for males and females. In most reports from the rest of the world papillary tumours predominate (*Winship* 1958). The exceptions are Uganda (*Templeton* 1973) and Colombia (*Cuello* 1969) where follicular carcinomas predominate. This study demonstrates a marked preponderance of follicular carcinomas.

Of the 68 cases, 36 were follicular (31 females) 24 papillary (19 females) 5 medullary (4 females) and 3 anaplastic (1 female). The age distribution conforms to that observed in other parts of the world with a preponderance of follicular carcinomas in the older age groups. The mean age of the patients with follicular carcinoma was 53 years and that with papillary carcinoma 40 years. There was a singular absence of thyroid carcinoma in children, not one case being found below the age of 20 years.

Follicular carcinoma appears to arise in most instances from a pre-existing nodule, whether this be a solitary adenoma or part of a multinodular goitre. Anaplastic carcinomas appear to develop from pre-existing follicular carcinomas.

Other Endocrine Glands

Because of the comparative rarity of tumours of other endocrine glands, age specific incidence rates could not be calculated.

Adrenal Gland: There were five cases of adrenal cortical adenoma – three males and two females varying in age from 36–80 years. There were five cases of adrenal cortical carcinoma – four males and one female varying in age from 16–67 years.

Phaeochromocytoma: Four cases were found – 3 females and one male varying in age from 26–55 years.

Pituitary Gland: All the tumours of the pituitary gland were chromophobe adenomas. There were 14 cases – 8 females and 6 males, the ages varying from 19–70 years.

Parathyroid Gland: Tumours of the parathyroid gland were remarkably rare, the ten year survey yielding only one adenoma.

Tumours of the Jaw

In the series of *Higginson* and *Oettle* (1960) ameloblastomas were observed in Blacks in 0.6% of all cancers as compared with 0.07% in Whites and 0.15% in Negroes in the United States. Similar findings have been reported from Uganda (*Davies* and *Davies* 1960; *Dodge* 1965). In Uganda (*Dodge* 1965) ameloblastomas, ossifying fibromas and antral carcinomas were the commonest encountered. However, several authors have questioned the apparent high incidence of jaw tumours in Africa and have suggested that the increase may be due in part to harvesting of a tumour with a long natural history (*Anand* et al. 1967; *Slavin* and *Cameron* 1969; *Mosadomi* 1975). *Mosadomi* (1975) claims that conclusions were reached in Africa without an adequate basis in most cases and it is still not possible to determine accurately the incidence of tumours in most African countries. He also claims that there is no clear racial predilection and one can explain the high incidence in Africa on the harvesting theory, the basis of which is that in cases of gross oro-facial tumours it is easier for neighbours or relatives to urge those afflicted to seek treatment and in addition with a slow growing painless lesion which does not endanger life, the cases accumulate until surgical facilities become available for their treatment.

Table 6.8. Tumours of the jaw

Fibrous dysplasia	17
Cementoma	9
Ameloblastoma	25
Myxoma	2
Adenomatoid odontogenic tumour	2
Complex odontoma	1
Pindborg tumour	1
Chondroblastoma	1
Osteogenic sarcoma	4
Chondrosarcoma	2
Miscellanous	2
Total	66

Table 6.9. Hodgkin's disease type subtype distribution and M:F ratios. *LP* Lymphocyte predominant; *NS* nodular sclerosing; *MC* mixed cellularity; *LD* lymphocyte depleted

	Male					Female			
Ages	LP	NS	MC	LD	M:F	LP	NS	MC	LD
0–14	11.8%	13.6%	54.9%	19.6%	1.8:1	10%	15%	60%	15%
15–39	4.9%	18.1%	55.5%	21.4%	3.5:1	5.8%	17.3%	57.7%	19.9%
40+	5.5%	18.2%	65.4%	11.8%	1.5:1	12.2%	12.2%	51.1%	24.4%

Benign lesions in this population have been well described by *Schmaman* et al. (1970). In the present study no clear distinction was drawn between fibrous dysplasia and ossifying fibroma. The survey yielded 66 cases (Table 6.8). The interpretation of these findings is uncertain. No comparison can be made with other population groups as the statistics available generally include all jaw lesions including benign cysts and antral carcinomas. *Shear* (1977) has recently presented figures to show that ameloblastoma is very much more common in Blacks than Whites, whereas dentigenrous cysts are much more common in Whites.

Hodgkin's Disease

Five hundred and fifty-seven Black subjects with a diagnosis of Hodgkin's disease were studied – 420 males and 137 females, M:F ratio of 3:1, and classified according to the Rye histological subtypes (*Lukes* et al. 1966) (Table 6.9). Of the 557 there were 88 children under the age of 15 years (15%), 347 (62%) were between 15 and 39 years and 122 (23%) over 40 years (*Vianna* et al. 1977).

Hodgkin's disease in Johannesburg thus shares the features recorded from elsewhere in the continent of Africa; the high frequency in childhood, the predominance of the mixed cellularity and lymphocyte depleted subtypes of poor prognosis evident in all age groups, and the paucity of cases of lymphocyte predominant and nodular sclerosing. However, an interesting feature, to which attention has been drawn elsewhere in Africa is that the nodular sclerosing form of Hodgkin's disease is a disease of males, unlike Caucasians where it is a disease mainly of young adult females. While in Blacks the predominant subtype is the mixed cellularity, it should be noted that there is, at all ages a high frequency of the lymphoid depleted subtype of Hodgkin's disease, again a feature noted elsewhere.

Thus in the high frequency in childhood and the gross male predominance, as well as in the disproportionate number of cases with poor histologic reactions, the population studied exhibits the features characteristic of Hodgkin's disease in non-affluent populations (*Correa* and *O'Conor* 1971; *Olisa* et al. 1977).

Conclusions

The ten year survey of malignant disease at Baragwanath Hospital is far from complete. Several organs have been omitted, notably *pancreas and biliary tract.* The reasons for this are obvious. The pathological diagnosis of pancreatic and biliary tract carcinoma is not only fraught with difficulty but is not that frequently made. Many pancreatic carcinomas are labelled with this diagnosis on clinical grounds, and therefore cannot be included in a study based on histological examination. A detailed analysis of all lymphomas has not yet been performed, nor is there any assessment of tumours of bone and soft tissues. Leukaemia is not included in the study, and no separate assessment was carried out of cancers in childhood. Eye tumours were also not analysed.

The accuracy of the population assessment of Soweto may be questioned. This is a very rough assessment, the figures, if anything, being an underestimate of the true population.

Several observations are worth reiterating. The squamous carcinomas of the upper gastrointestinal tract and the hypopharynx are all without exception, tumours predominantly of males over the age of 40 years. Table 6.10 demonstrates the male: female ratio of carcinoma of the larynx, tongue, mouth, tonsil and oesophagus. In every instance the percentage of males is over 80% and in four of the five tumours the percentage of males is over 90%.

Apart from tumours of the oesophagus and liver, the Black male has a much smaller cancer problem than his Caucasian counterpart. Similarly, apart from carcinoma of the cervix, the Black female does not have a major cancer problem.

Oesophageal carcinoma apart, gastrointestinal cancers are rare in the Black population. A twenty year survey of carcinoma of the large bowel has not shown any significant increase despite the process of urbanization and Westernization. The twenty year period, may however, be too short for any changes. In general, no significant alteration in the incidence of any tumour was seen during the ten year period of the survey except for an inordinately high number of prostatic carcinomas in the last year of the survey. The significance of this finding is uncertain.

Breast cancer has a low incidence with poor therapeutic results. The reason for the latter is the late presentation for therapy and not more aggressive tumours. Carcinoma of the cervix has a very high incidence. Chorionepithelioma does not have a high incidence compared with other population groups and endometrial and ovarian carcinoma continue to be rare. Tumours of the male genitourinary system are infrequent. Testicular tumours and transitional cell tumours of the urinary tract are seldom seen. There were only two cases of transitional cell tumour of the renal pelvis. The curious distribution of malignant melanoma is confirmed, in which 80% arise in the lower

Table 6.10. Male–female ratio of carcinomas of the larynx, tongue, mouth, tonsil and oesophagus

	Total	Males	Females	%Males
Larynx	186	175	11	94
Tongue	115	106	9	92
Mouth	89	83	6	93
Tonsil	37	35	2	94
Oesophagus	1331	1110	221	93
Average	1758	1509	249	85

Table 6.11. Average annual incidence per 100,000 – all ages – Nigeria

	Males		Females
Squamous carcinoma of the tongue	0.1		0.1
Squamous carcinoma of cheek and mouth	0.4		0.3
Salivary gland tumours (males and females)		0.8	
Squamous carcinoma of the oesophagus	0.3		0.3
Hepatocellular carcinoma	4.9		1.6
Squamous carcinoma of the stomach	2.4		2.1
Carcinoma of the rectum	0.6		0.7
Carcinoma of the colon	0.4		0.5
Squamous carcinoma of the antrum	0.7		0.5
Squamous carcinoma of the larynx	0.4		0.1
Carcinoma of the breast (females)	–		5.8
Squamous carcinoma of the cervix	–		7.0
Carcinoma of the endometrium	–		0.5
Chorionepithelioma	–		2.51
Tumours of the ovary	–		3.0
Carcinoma of the prostate	1.8		–
Tumours of the testis	0.2		–
Squamous carcinoma of the penis	0.1		–
Malignant tumours of the kidney (males and females)		0.35	
Carcinoma of the bladder	0.9		0.7
Malignant melanoma of the skin	0.3		0.7
Tumours of the central nervous system (males and females)		0.40	
Carcinoma of the thyroid	0.3		1.0

limb, an area that is comparatively hypopigmented. Tumours of the central nervous and endocrine systems are infrequent.

The high incidence of nephroblastoma can be ascribed to subjects from more remote areas coming to Baragwanath Hospital for treatment. The question may well be posed whether this does not apply to other tumours as well. This seems unlikely and would not appear to be a major factor in influencing the statistics, and would in any event merely enhance their significance.

The figures presented here are vastly different from those in Blacks in the United States, whose incidence rates approximate those of the White population. These findings indicate that in most instances the factors responsible for the differences are environmental. The one exception is testicular tumours which show a low incidence in Blacks throughout the world, suggesting a genetic basis for their rarity.

Tables 6.11–6.15 show the comparative age specific incidence rates for tumours in Nigeria, Denmark, Wales and England, California Blacks, and California Whites.

Summary

A 10 year survey of malignant disease at Baragwanath Hospital showed that apart from tumours of the oesophagus and liver, the Black male has a much smaller cancer problem than his Caucasian counterpart. Similarly, apart from carcinoma of the cervix, the Black female does not have a major cancer problem. Oesophageal carcinoma apart,

Table 6.12. Average annual incidence per 100,000 – all ages – Denmark

	Males		Females
Squamous carcinoma of the tongue	0.5		0.5
Squamous carcinoma of cheek and mouth	1.0		0.9
Salivary gland tumours (males and females)		1.3	
Squamous carcinoma of the oesophagus	4.3		2.5
Hepatocellular carcinoma	4.4		3.2
Squamous carcinoma of the stomach	32.8		21.8
Carcinoma of the rectum	23.8		17.2
Carcinoma of the colon	23.0		28.2
Squamous carcinoma of the antrum	1.3		0.7
Squamous carcinoma of the larynx	4.6		0.7
Carcinoma of the breast (females)	–		105.3
Squamous carcinoma of the cervix	–		37.9
Carcinoma of the endometrium	–		16.5
Chorionepithelioma	–		0.0
Tumours of the ovary	–		20.9
Carcinoma of the prostate	32.8		–
Tumours of the testis	5.0		–
Squamous carcinoma of the penis	1.4		–
Malignant tumours of the kidney (males and females)		7.0	
Carcinoma of the bladder	22.9		6.8
Malignant melanoma of the skin	3.5		6.0
Tumours of the central nervous system			
Carcinoma of the thyroid	1.0		2.6

Table 6.13. Average annual incidence per 100,000 – all ages – Wales and England

	Males		Females
Squamous carcinoma of the tongue	1.4		0.9
Squamous carcinoma of cheek and mouth	2.2		1.2
Salivary gland tumours (males and females)		1.4	
Squamous carcinoma of the oesophagus	9.3		8.3
Hepatocellular carcinoma	2.0		1.1
Squamous carcinoma of the stomach	39.0		26.3
Carcinoma of the rectum	20.6		18.9
Carcinoma of the colon	23.0		30.5
Squamous carcinoma of the antrum	1.2		0.9
Squamous carcinoma of the larynx	6.2		1.2
Carcinoma of the breast (females)	–		69.0
Squamous carcinoma of the cervix	–		20.0
Carcinoma of the endometrium	–		13.7
Chorionepithelioma	–		0.0
Tumours of the ovary	–		15.0
Carcinoma of the prostate	24.3		–
Tumours of the testis	2.3		–
Squamous carcinoma of the penis	1.1		–
Malignant tumours of the kidney (males and females)		4.3	
Carcinoma of the bladder	20.4		6.9
Malignant melanoma of the skin	1.1		2.6
Tumours of the central nervous system		6.6	
Carcinoma of the thyroid	0.8		1.9

Table 6.14. Average annual incidence per 100,000 – all ages – California Blacks

	Males		Females
Squamous carcinoma of the tongue	1.7		1.3
Squamous carcinoma of cheek and mouth	4.1		1.3
Salivary gland tumours (males and females)		1.1	
Squamous carcinoma of the oesophagus	12.1		3.5
Hepatocellular carcinoma	3.4		1.3
Squamous carcinoma of the stomach	16.6		5.3
Carcinoma of the rectum	8.1		6.7
Carcinoma of the colon	17.9		17.4
Squamous carcinoma of the antrum	0.6		0.4
Squamous carcinoma of the larynx	9.6		1.3
Carcinoma of the breast (females)	–		74.6
Squamous carcinoma of the cervix	–		23.7
Carcinoma of the endometrium	–		11.2
Chorionepithelioma	–		0.4
Tumours of the ovary	–		8.3
Carcinoma of the prostate	51.9		–
Tumours of the testis	1.0		–
Squamous carcinoma of the penis	1.0		–
Malignant tumours of the kidney (males and females)		3.25	
Carcinoma of the bladder	6.7		3.5
Malignant melanoma of the skin	0.6		0.6
Tumours of the central nervous system		3.9	
Carcinoma of the thyroid	1.5		2.5

Table 6.15. Average annual incidence per 100,000 – all ages – California Whites

	Males		Females
Squamous carcinoma of the tongue	3.8		2.1
Squamous carcinoma of cheek and mouth	5.0		3.2
Salivary gland tumours (males and females)		1.2	
Squamous carcinoma of the oesophagus	4.8		2.9
Hepatocellular carcinoma	3.3		2.0
Squamous carcinoma of the stomach	14.2		9.5
Carcinoma of the rectum	18.3		16.1
Carcinoma of the colon	34.6		38.5
Squamous carcinoma of the antrum	0.7		0.6
Squamous carcinoma of the larynx	8.7		1.6
Carcinoma of the breast (females)	–		52.0
Squamous carcinoma of the cervix	–		14.6
Carcinoma of the endometrium	–		39.4
Chorionepithelioma	–		0.2
Tumours of the ovary	–		18.0
Carcinoma of the prostate	56.0		–
Tumours of the testis	4.8		–
Squamous carcinoma of the penis	0.8		–
Malignant tumours of the kidney (males and females)		5.2	
Carcinoma of the bladder	23.3		8.3
Malignant melanoma of the skin	7.0		7.7
Tumours of the central nervous system (males and females)		6.6	
Carcinoma of the thyroid	3.0		7.0

gastrointestinal cancers are rare in the Black population despite the process of urbanization and Westernization.

Since the completion of the survey there has been an inordinate number of prostatic carcinomas. This parallels what has happened to the American Negro since the early 1940's.

The poor therapeutic results in breast carcinoma are due to late presentation for therapy and not because of a more aggressive type of tumour.

The curious distribution of malignant melanomas is confirmed, in which 80% of these tumours arise in the lower limb, an area that is comparatively hypopigmented.

Note Added in Proof

Recent studies have lent further weight to the oncogenic role of hepatitis B virus (*Kew* et al. 1979, 1980; *Kew* 1981; *Shafritz* and *Kew* 1981; *Shafritz* et al. 1981). *Isaacson* et al. (1979) have however shown a marked difference in the surface antigen positivity in cases from Baragwanath Hospital compared with subjects from Mozambique, and very recently *Paterson* and *Isaacson* (1982) in a study of hepatocellular carcinoma during the periods 1956–1960 and 1976–1980 have shown evidence of a significant increase in the overall average age, in the proportion of female cases, while the percentage of HBSAg positive cases has fallen.

Chapter 7

Neurotrophic Feet

Idiopathic Neurotrophic Feet in Blacks

Idiopathic neurotrophic feet in Blacks is a well known clinical entity (*Perdikis* and *Bremner* 1969; *Trope* and *Crookes* 1975). It is generally referred to by the descriptive term "vrot foot" which describes the decayed appearance of the neglected feet when first seen, characterized by ulceration of the sole of the foot in the region of the metatarsal heads, painless destruction of the bones of the feet and a peripheral neuropathy (Fig. 7.1). Usually no cause can be found. All the patients thus far reported have been males generally below the age of 50 years. Most were considered heavy drinkers and in most instances this takes the form of home brewed alcoholic beverages. Clinically, there is often a perforating ulcer on the undersurface of the foot with evidence of bony resorption and clawing. Most cases show a shortening of the toes and in some there are just stubbs remaining. This change is supposedly due to infection with osteolysis and absorption and also due to the neuropathy which apparently induces increased vascularity of the bone with resultant rarefraction. With progressive neuropathy there

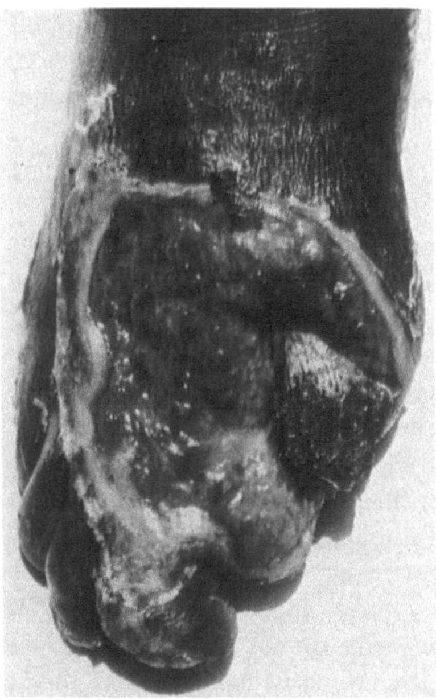

Fig. 7.1. Typical clinical appearance of idiopathic neurotrophic feet

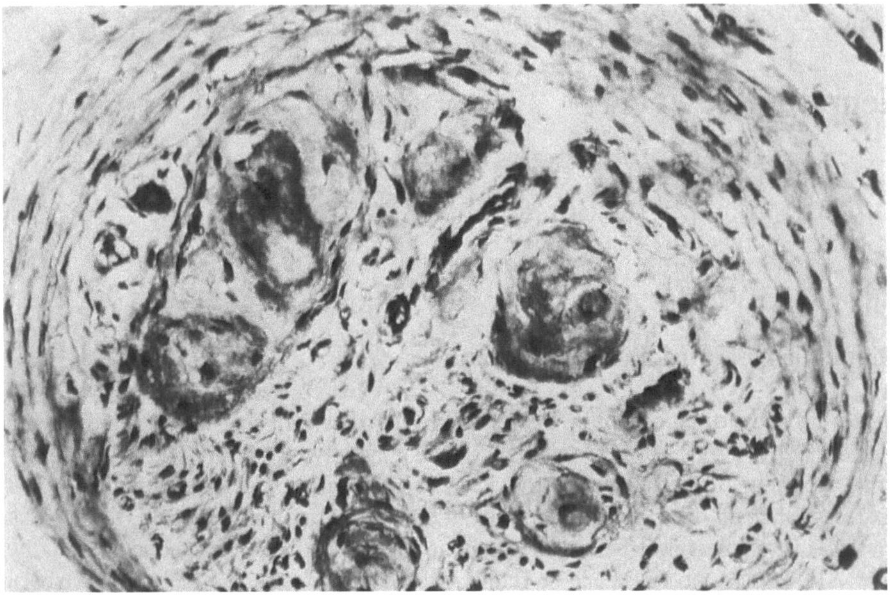

Fig. 7.2. Areas of globular hyalinization in a nerve fibre. Elastic-Masson, ×280

is eventually extension at the metatarso-phalangeal joints and flexion at the interphalangeal joints. The metatarsal head is pushed through the skin of the ball of the foot resulting in the perforating ulcer. A number of cases also have clinical pellagra. In nearly all cases no evidence of a vascular deficit has been found, but there is generally a neurological deficit affecting mainly light touch, pain and temperature. *Perdikis* and *Bremner* (1969) and *Trope* and *Crookes* (1975) suggest that the condition is the result of excessive ingestion of alcohol resulting in central and peripheral nerve degeneration. Clinically, the lesion is similar to diabetic neuropathy and the primary presentation is that of a peripheral neuropathy.

All the studies, including angiography, do not point to a vascular deficit, and histologically in all instances the striking finding is gross demyelinization, with evidence of axonal degeneration (*Isaacson* 1977). Some nerves undergo a globular hyaline degeneration, and in advanced cases there is perineural fibrosis. A diffuse neuropathy is present in which the pathogenesis is that of gross demyelinization similar to that observed in diabetic neuropathy (Figs. 7.2–7.4).

Surprising vascular changes are also a fairly constant finding. The large blood vessels are always patent and there is no suggestion of atherosclerosis or Buerger's disease, and the changes are confined to the smaller distal digital blood vessels which are increased in number and filled with blood. This latter finding may be so prominent as to mimic a "tumour blush" radiologically (Fig. 7.5). Pathologically, this is represented by a marked increase in the number of small blood vessels including arterioles and capillaries, although the increase may not be real but may reflect dilatation and prominence of existing blood vessels (Fig. 7.6). In addition the small arteries and arterioles show marked thickening of their walls particularly of the intima with hyperplasia of the

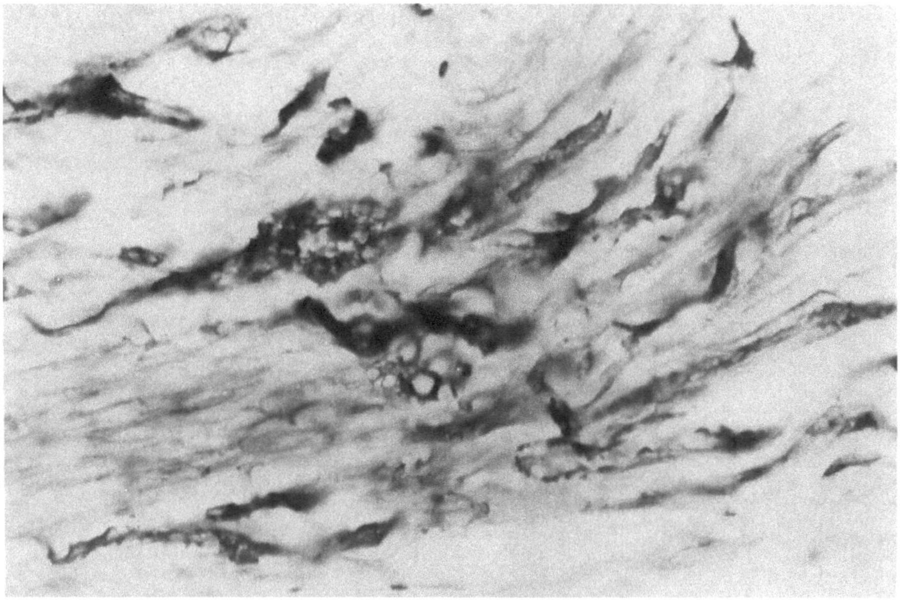

Fig. 7.3. Normal myelin from a control nerve. Luxol fast blue, × 700

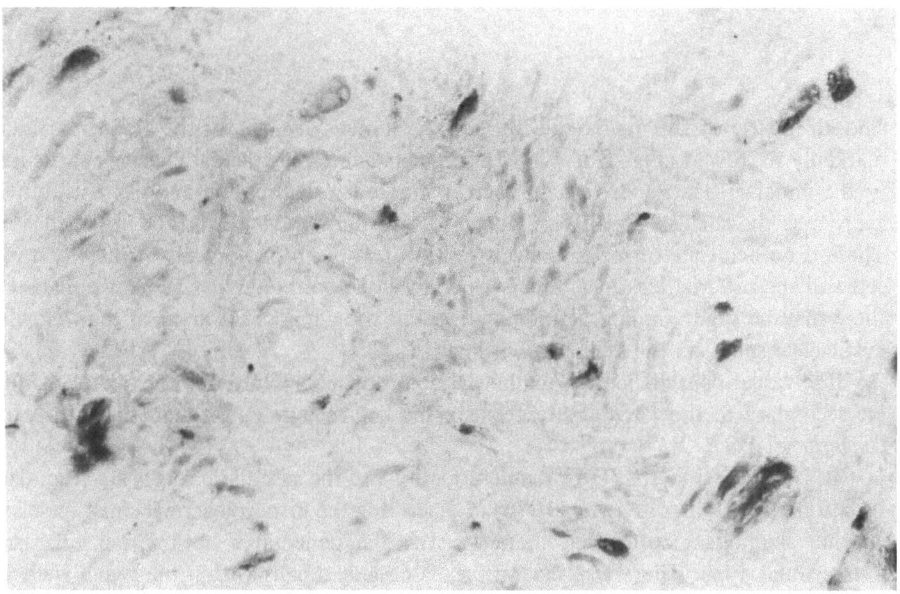

Fig. 7.4. Nerve from case of idiopathic neurotrophic feet showing complete demyelinization. Luxol fast blue, × 700

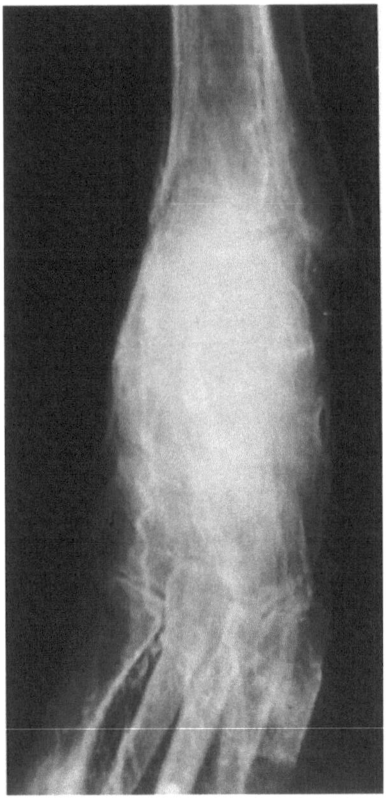

Fig. 7.5. Apparent increased vascularization in the foot. (By courtesy of Dr. *D. Miller*)

smooth muscle of the media and intima. The lumens of many of the blood vessels are markedly narrowed (Figs. 7.7, 7.8). In some instances the vascular changes, particularly the endarteritis, are present in foci of marked inflammation and necrosis, but in every case the changes are also present in sections far removed from the inflamed sites. There is no evidence of inflammatory cell infiltration into the walls of the blood vessels and the internal elastic lamina is generally intact, although in one or two instances there may be slight fraying. Some blood vessels show marked oedema of the wall with cystic clear spaces in the media and intima (Fig. 7.9).

The vasculitis is difficult to explain. It does not seem likely that the neural changes are secondary to the vascular alterations as has been suggested for diabetic neuropathy (*Fagerberg*1959).

It seems possible that both the neuropathy and the vascular changes are secondary to chronic alcoholism. *Factor* (1976) in describing the intramyocardial small vessels in chronic alcoholism noted that there was vascular oedema of both intracellular and extracellular type. There was separation of individual cells within the vessel walls by clear spaces. Perivascular fibrosis was prominent and many of the vessels showed striking intimal proliferation with oedema and medial sclerosis. Major narrowing of the lumen was seen when the sclerosis affected the entire vessel wall in a symmetrical

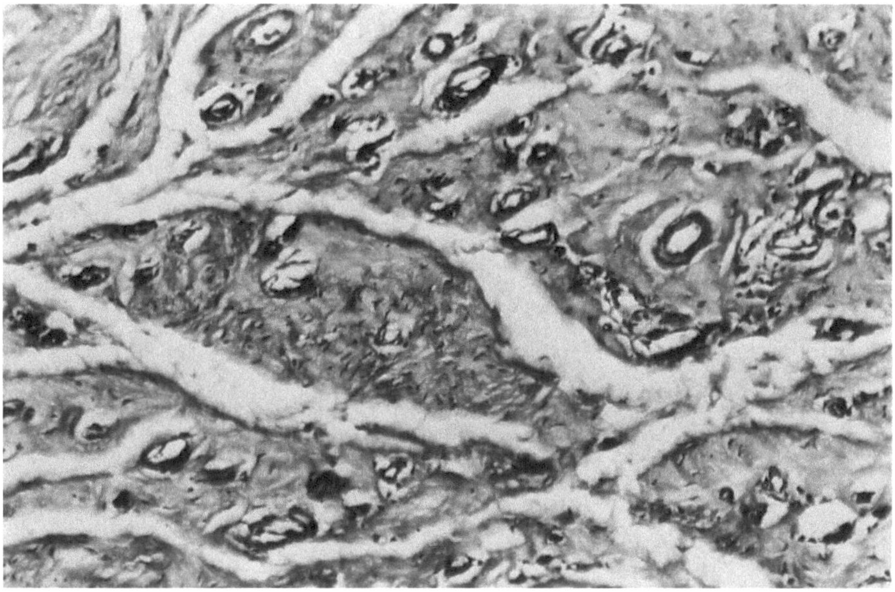

Fig. 7.6. Dilatation and prominence of small blood vessels in the foot. H&E, × 175

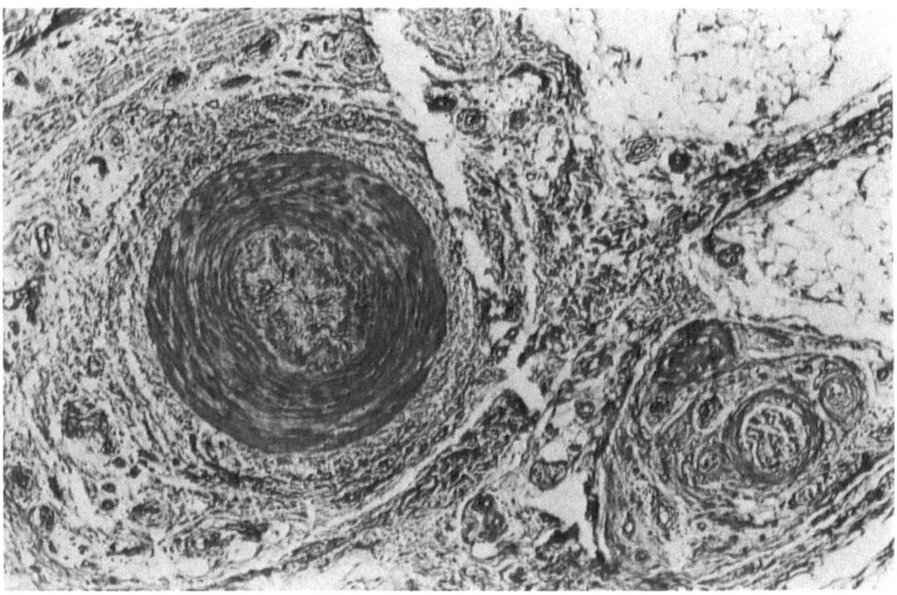

Fig. 7.7. Endarteritis of small artery almost occluding the lumen; note perineural fibrosis at bottom right. Elastic-Masson, × 70

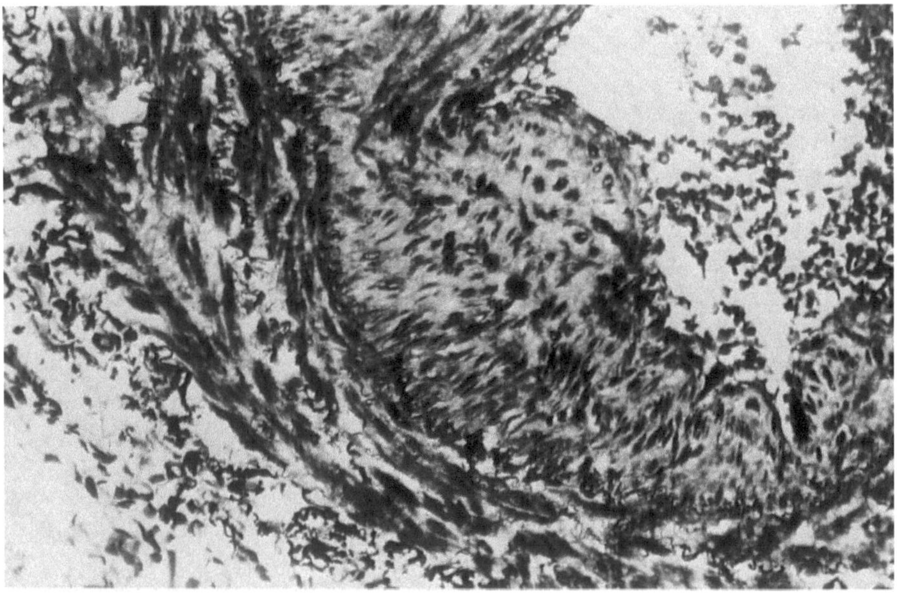

Fig. 7.8. Marked hyperplasia of the smooth muscle of intima and media. Elastic-Masson, ×280

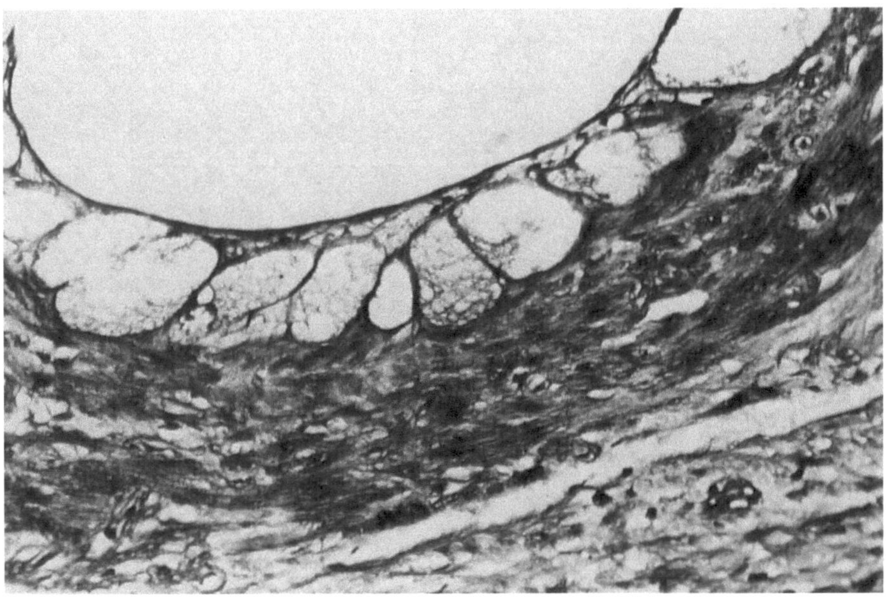

Fig. 7.9. Artery showing cystic clear spaces in the media and intima due to oedema fluid. H&E, ×280

fashion. The sclerosis was often asymmetric. In some instances the internal elastic lamina was disrupted and duplicated. It is however, of interest to note that despite these marked vascular changes in the hearts of chronic alcoholics, clinically, these patients had never had any cardiac symptoms.

Experimental data suggest that oedema in the vessel wall is secondary to endothelial cell damage, widening of intercellular gaps and diffusion of plasma into the vascular wall. *Pintar* et al. (1965) reported essentially similar findings in the hearts of chronic alcoholics. In contrast to the large and medium sized branches, the walls of the small branches of the coronary arteries were arranged in less organised layers with an increase of collagen in the adventitia. It is possible that subjects with idiopathic neurotrophic feet are chronic alcoholics who develop a peripheral neuropathy which accounts for the clinical symptomatology, but that, in addition, a vasculitis is present affecting the distal arteries and arterioles, the vascular alterations also being produced by chronic alcoholism.

Alcohol consumption is of importance in this disease. Of the 15 cases reported by *Trope* and *Crookes* (1975), 13 admitted to being heavy drinkers and 2 to light alcohol consumption. Many of their subjects had no homes of their own and lived in hostels, environments that predispose to heavy drinking. *Bureau* and *Barriere* (1958) reported a series of cases of "ulcerating and mutilating trophic lesions of the lower limbs". They described 26 men and 1 woman, all adults varying in age from 30 to 56 years who were all severely addicted to alcohol, and who presented with perforating ulcers and a progressive deformity of the whole foot. Changes were not observed in the upper limbs. In their cases arteriography of the small vessels of the legs showed arteriovenous communications producing tufts, the number of which was proportional to the severity and duration of ulcerated lesions.

Summary

The condition of idiopathic neurotrophic feet in Blacks is characterized by a decayed appearance of the feet with ulceration of the sole in the region of the metatarsal heads, painless destruction of the bones of the feet and peripheral neuropathy. The salient pathological features are those of gross demyelinization and marked changes in the distal blood vessels. The vascular changes include medial and intimal hypertrophy with luminal narrowing, although clinically the limbs do not show evidence of poor blood supply. It is suggested that both the neural and the vascular changes are secondary to chronic alcoholism.

Chapter 8

Perinatal Mortality

Barawanath Hospital serves a large Black community in which there is malnutrition, ignorance and inadequate antenatal care. Owing to the inherent shape of the pelvis of the black female, there are a large number of cases of cephalo–pelvic disproportion which are rarely seen in more highly developed communities. As a result there are a large number of stillbirths, premature deliveries and neonatal deaths. These factors should theoretically produce a high incidence of cerebral birth injury (*Shnier* and *Isaacson* 1965).

In 1979 *Stein* and *Mouton* carried out an autopsy study on 103 neonates who died during a five month period. Of the 103 autopsies 84 were on singletons and 19 on twins. The causes of death in singletons are listed in Table 8.1. There were an undue number of twins, thus confirming the greater vulnerability of babies born of multiple pregnancy.

Among both singletons and twins, neonates who were preterm and AGA (appropriate for gestational age) constituted the largest group (43%). This far exceeds the overall incidence of such babies (7%). A somewhat smaller group were preterm babies who were SGA (small for gestational age) (25%); in all, the incidence of babies of low

Table 8.1. Causes of death in singletons (*Stein* and *Mouton* 1979)

Cause of death	Number	
Extrinsic perinatal hypoxia (including meconium aspiration)		29
Respiratory distress syndrome		23
Infections		19
Pneumonia	11	
Meningitis	3	
Septicaemia	3	
Syphilis	2	
Congenital anomalies		6
Myelomeningocele	2	
Duodenal atresia	1	
Hypoplastic lungs	1	
Hypoplastic lungs and dysplastic kidneys	1	
Thanatophoric dwarfism	1	
Birth trauma – cerebral haemorrhage		3
Necrotizing enterocolitis		2
Kernicterus		1

birth weight was (72%). This is keeping with most findings that these babies are the largest category of the 'newborn-at-risk'. In the overall neonatal population, the incidence of low-birth-weight babies is 20% (*Stein* and *Ellis* 1974). The majority of deaths occurred on the first day of life (60%); in all more than 90% died in the first week. This high incidence in the first week confirms the view that most of the problems stem from poor antenatal attendance and are predominantly of socio-economic origin. The commonest cause of death in their series was extrinsic perinatal hypoxia (36%) including intra and extra uterine asphyxia with or without meconium aspiration. The largest category here was the SGA group with the attendant background of placental insufficiency, again reflecting the high incidence of dysmaturity in this population. Respiratory distress syndrome accounted for 30% of the deaths, all in low birth weight babies markedly preterm and AGA. As in the previous survey (*Shnier* and *Isaacson* 1965) most of these occurred within the first 24 hours.

Pulmonary haemorrhage was a very rare cause of death in this series, although it was relatively common in the previous series (*Shnier* and *Isaacson* 1965). Pulmonary haemorrhage is often the fatal manifestation of hypothermia and in recent years, with better care of both the hospital-born group and those born before arrival at hospital, this has become much less of a problem. Sclerema, which is another manifestation of hypothermia and which was common place, particularly among low-birth-weight babies 2–3 decades ago, is hardly seen at all now.

Infection was the cause of death in 19%. The majority of deaths occurred in preterm babies; thus showing their vulnerability to infection.

Birth trauma was a relatively rare cause of death (4%) as in the previous study by *Shnier* and *Isaacson* (1965). Respiratory distress syndrome was a much commoner cause of death than would have been anticipated on clinical grounds. This appears to be due to the fact that these deaths occurred particularly early – the majority before 18 hours, and possibly before the full blown clinical picture became manifest.

Thus the commonest cause of death was asphyxia, probably associated with the high incidence of SGA infants seen and possibly associated with varying degrees of placental insufficiency.

Kwashiorkor

There is a remarkably consistent pattern of change in cases of severe kwashiorkor in childhood (*Trowell* et al. 1954). The pancreas, lymphoid tissue, salivary glands, lacrimal glands, thyroid and the small intestine all undergo atrophic changes (Figs. 8.1–8.4). There is wasting of the muscles. The liver shows marked fatty change (Fig. 8.5). *Trowell* et al. (1954) described a fine fibrosis of the liver appearing after a very prolonged period, but no one has confirmed this observation, and there is certainly no evidence that the fatty liver of kwashiorkor progresses to cirrhosis or even increased portal tract fibrosis. Subjects with kwashiorkor either recover completely or die (*Stein* and *Isaacson* 1960). It is however, possible that the patient who has recovered from kwashiorkor may be more susceptible in adult life to other noxious influences affecting the liver.

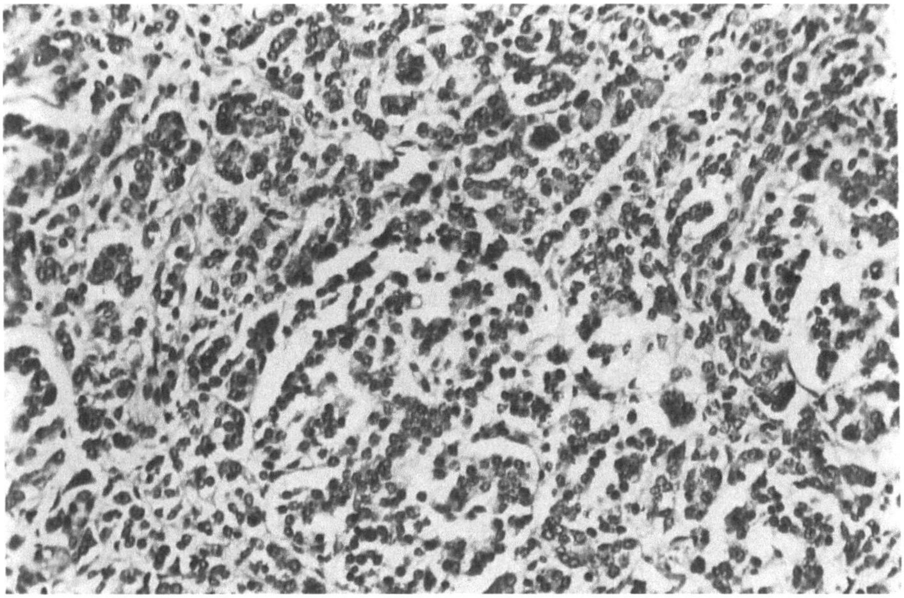

Fig. 8.1. Severe acinar atrophy of pancreas. Islet of Langerhans is present in the centre of the photomicrograph. H&E, ×280

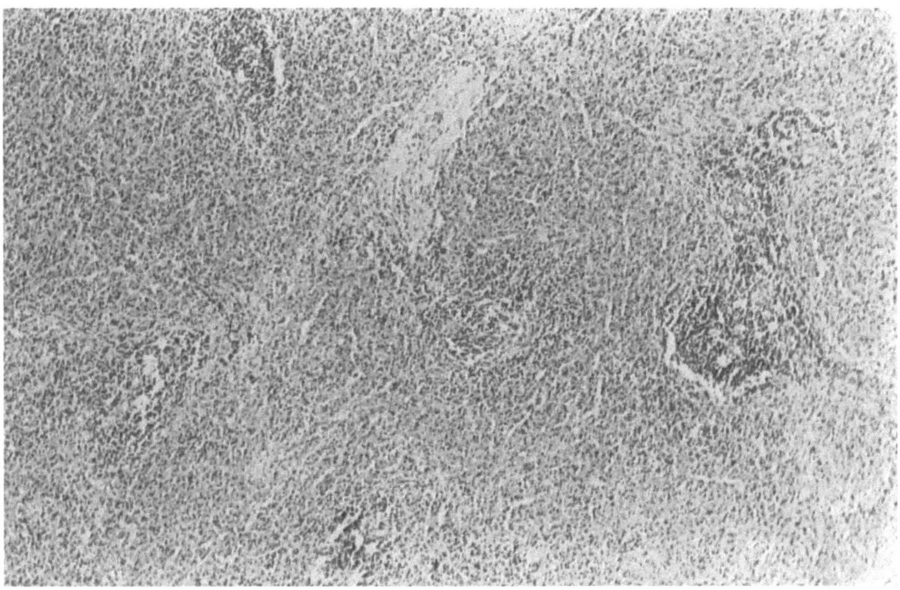

Fig. 8.2. Section of spleen showing atrophy of malphigian corpuscles in keeping with the generalized atrophy of lymphoid tissue. H&E, ×70

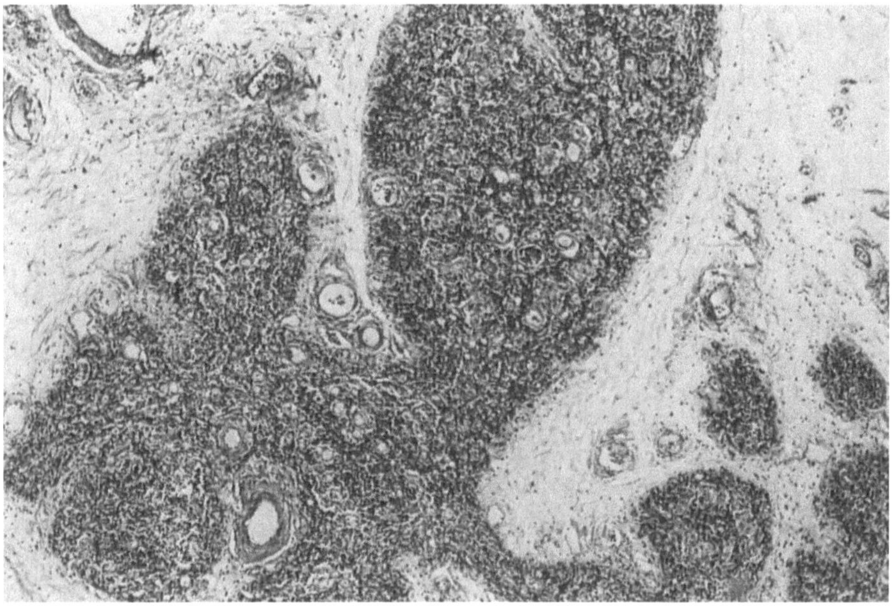

Fig. 8.3. Section of thymus showing marked atrophy. H&E, ×70

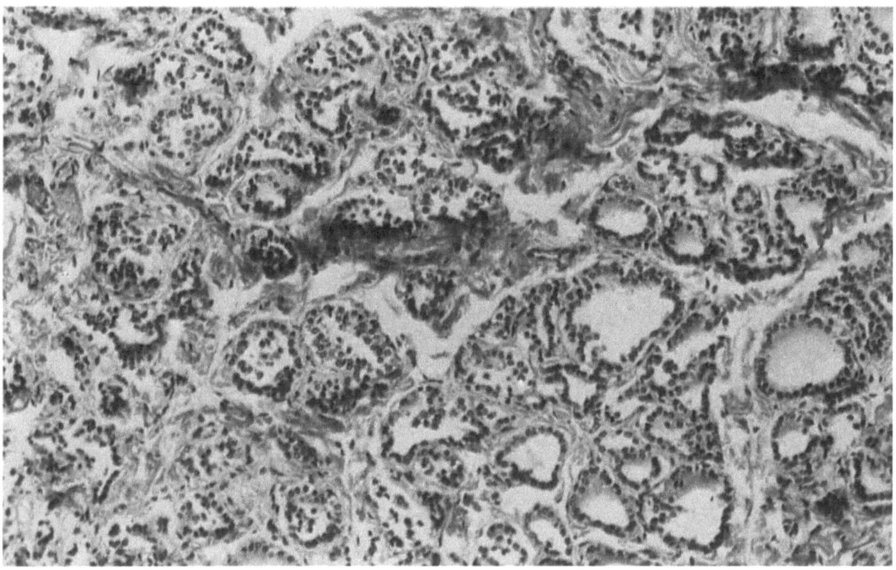

Fig. 8.4. Section of thyroid showing atrophy with diminution of colloid and flattening of the follicular lining cells. H&E, ×175

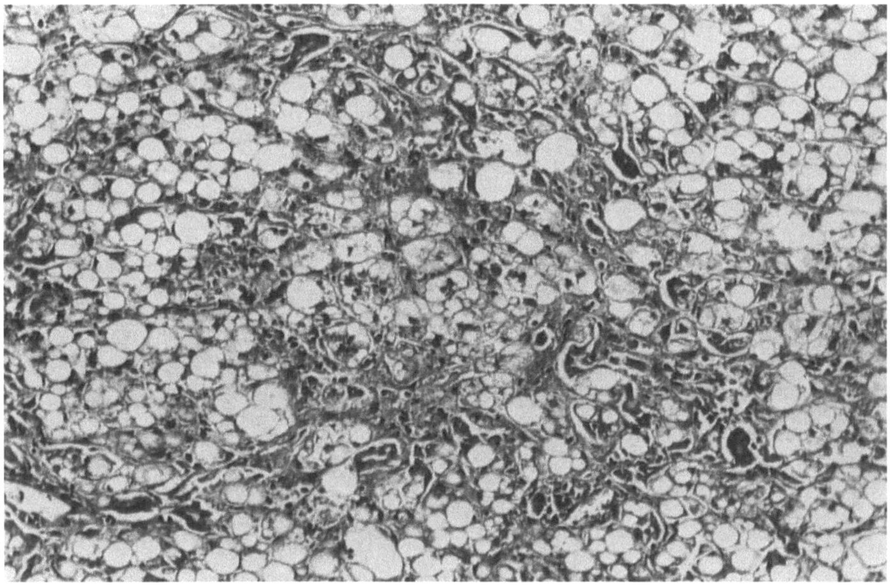

Fig. 8.5. Severe fatty change of liver in kwashiorkor. H&E, ×175

Many subjects with kwashiorkor show multivisceral fatty change and it may be impossible to distinguish these cases from those of Reye's syndrome. In some cases considerable quantities of fat may be observed in the kidneys particularly in the proximal convoluted tubules (Fig. 8.6). Aflatoxin may be of importance in hepatocarcinogenesis in this population (*Van Rensburg* et al. 1975). *Olson* et al. (1971) have shown that aflatoxin may play a role in the causation of Reye's syndrome in Thailand, a condition in which hepatic steatosis is an important feature. There is no doubt that protein malnutrition alone can cause the severe hepatic steatosis of kwashiorkor, but other factors such as aflatoxin may aggravate the fatty change seen in these children. In fact, recent, as yet unpublished observations have shown high levels of aflatoxin in the livers of numbers of children dying of kwashiorkor.

The cardiac changes in kwashiorkor are not well defined. *Wharton* et al. (1969) described radiological changes of an increase in the cardiothoracic ratio, with evidence of increased left ventricular voltage in the electrocardiogram. Changes in the T-wave pattern and histology suggested myocardial disease, and this was supported by raised levels of the first band of serum lactate dehydrogenase and a fall with nutritional repletion. They found the heart at autopsy to be paler than normal, with muscle fibres smaller than normal and separated from each other by oedematous stroma (Fig. 8.7). In some instances the fibres in the papillary muscles and in the subendocardial zone are vacuolated. The myocardium may show mild fatty infiltration and occasional foci of necrosis of fibres may be seen. However, these authors were the first to point out that the histological changes in the heart varied only in degree from those found in other Black children without kwashiorkor and that the lesions may be non-specific.

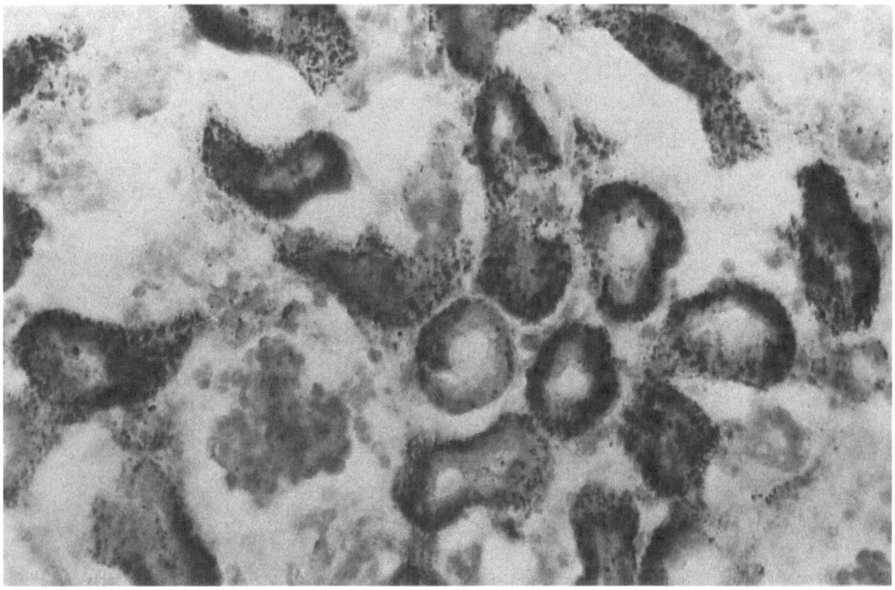

Fig. 8.6. High power view of lipid positive material in proximal convoluted tubules. Oil red, × 420

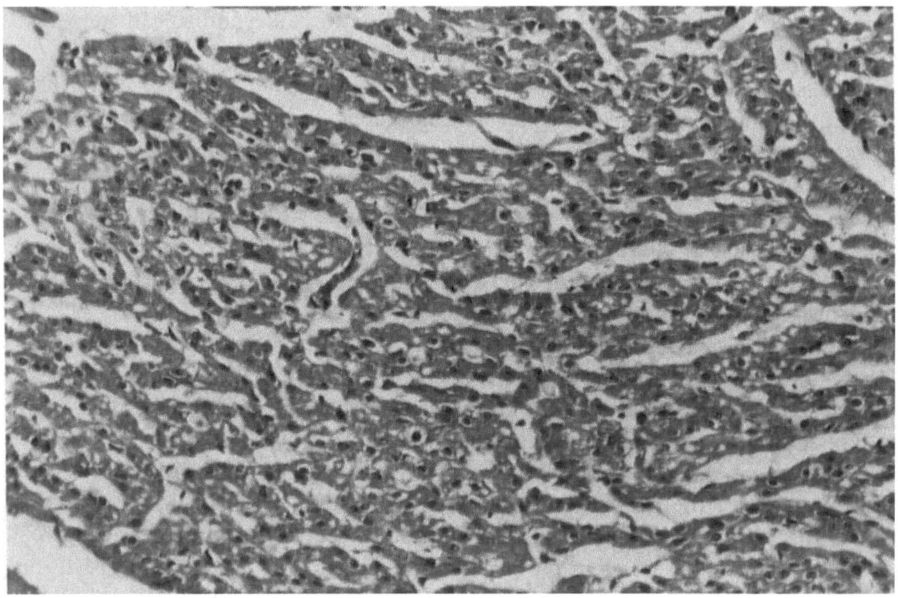

Fig. 8.7. Section of myocardium in case of kwashiorkor showing atrophy of the muscle fibres. H&E, × 280

In some instances the patients present in a low out-put state with cold extremities and a poor pulse volume (*Smythe* et al. 1962). Radiologically the hearts may be abnormally small. *Smythe* et al. (1962) suggest that some of the changes present are similar to those seen in idiopathic heart failure in adults (*Higginson* et al. 1960). Although rare, an occasional case with mural thrombi resembling idiopathic heart failure has been seen. It is possible that some idiopathic heart failures in adults may be the sequel of kwashiorkor in childhood (*Seftel* 1973).

Summary

Despite the high incidence of cephalopelvic disproportion, precipitate labour and other obstetrical abnormalities which predispose to cerebral birth trauma, 90% of the deaths in the perinatal period are due to gross pulmonary pathology including extrinsic perinatal hypoxia and intra and extra uterine axphyxia with or without meconium aspiration.

Kwashiorkor is extremely common in this population and is due to protein malnutrition. Other factors may aggravate the steatosis seen in these subjects and aflatoxin may be of importance in this context.

References

Chapter 1

Altman H, Stein H (1956) Idiopathic hypertrophy of the heart in African children. A report of four cases. Br Med J 1:1207–1210

Bada JL (1973) Idiopathic cardiomyopathy with particular reference to findings in Africa. S Afr Med J 47:570–575

Becker BJP, Chatgidakis CB, van Lingen B (1953) Cardiovascular collagenosis with parietal endocardial thrombosis: a clinicopathologic study of 40 cases. Circulation 7:345–356

Black-Schaffer B (1957) Infantile endocardial fibroelastosis. Arch Pathol 63:281–306

Brandt V, Keeley KJ, Metz J, Seftel H, Soldin P (1965) Red cell thiamine concentration in idiopathic cardiomyopathy. S Afr J Med Sci 30:64–66

Brigden W, Robinson J (1964) Alcoholic heart disease. Br Med J 2:1283–1289

Brockington IF, Olsen EGT, Goodwin JF (1967) Endomyocardial fibrosis in Europeans resident in Tropical Africa. Lancet 1:583–588

Connor DH, Somers K, Hutt MSR, Manion WC, D'Arbela PG (1968) Endomyocardial fibrosis in Uganda (Davies' disease) Part II. An epidemiologic, clinical and pathologic study. Am Heart J 75:108–124

Davies JNP (1948) Endocardial fibrosis in Africans. E Afr Med J 25:10–14

Davies JNP (1961) The heart of Africa (Cardiac pathology in the population of Uganda). Lab Invest 10:205–215

Edington GM, Jackson JG (1963) The pathology of heart muscle disease and endomyocardial fibrosis in Nigeria. J Pathol Bact 86:333–344

Emmanuel R (1972) Familial cardiomyopathies. Prostgrad Med J 48:742–745

Falase AO, Cole TO, Osuntokun BO (1973) Myocardial infarction in Nigerians. Trop Geogr Med 25:147–150

Gillanders AD (1951) Nutritional heart disease. Br Heart J 13:177–196

Grusin H (1957) Acute reversible heart failure in Africans. Circulation 16:27–35

Higginson J, Gillanders AD, Murray JF (1952) The heart in chronic malnutrition. Br Heart J 14:213–224

Higginson J, Isaacson C, Simson I (1960) The pathology of cryptogenic heart disease. Arch Pathol 70:497–507

Isaacson C (1977) The changing pattern of heart disease in South African Blacks. S Afr Med J 52:793–798

Kallichurum S (1976) The heart in cardiomyopathy, a postmortem study. S Afr Med J 50:1585–1591

MacPhail AP, Simon MO, Torrance JD, Bothwell TH, Isaacson C (1979) Changing patterns of dietary iron overload in Black South Africans. Am J Clin Nutr 32:1272–1278

Parry EOH, Abrahams DG (1965) The natural history of endomyocardial fibrosis. Q J Med 34:383–408

Powell SJ, Wright R (1965) Cardiomyopathy in Durban. S Afr Med J 39:1062–1066

Reid JVO (1970) Trial of tryptophan prophylaxis in patients liable to African cardiomyopathy. S Afr Med J 44:732–735
Seftel HC (1973) Cardiomyopathies in Johannesburg Bantu. S Afr Med J 47:321–324
Seftel HC, Metz J, Lakier JB (1972) Cardiomyopathies in Johannesburg Bantu – I Aetiology and characteristics of beri-beri heart disease. S Afr Med J 46:1707–1713
Shaper AG (1968) Cardiomegaly of unknown origin in South Africa. Trop Geogr Med 20:291–297
Smythe PM, Swanepoel A, Campbell JAH (1962) The heart in kwashiorkor. Br Med J 1:67–73
Stein H, Shnier MH, Wayburne S, Isaacson C (1964) Cardiomyopathy in African children. Arch Dis Child 39:610–617
Wharton BA, Balmer SE, Somers K, Templeton AC (1969) The myocardium in kwashiorkor. Q J Med 38:107–116

Chapter 2

Aderele WI, Seriki O (1974) Hypertension in Nigerian children. Arch Dis Child 49: 313–317
Akingkugbe OO (1969) A school survey of arterial pressure and proteinuria in Abadan Nigeria. East Afr Med J 46:257–261
Anderson M, Walker ARP, Lutz W, Higginson J (1959) Chemical and pathological studies on aortic atherosclerosis. Arch Pathol 68:380–391
Becker BJP (1946) Hypertensive heart disease. S Afr J Med Sci 11:107–120
Bertrand E, Aye H, Beda B, Barabe P, Lebras M, Delloue M (1974) Quelques aspects des coronarites observées á Abidjan chezdes Noirs Africains. Afr J Med Sci 2:217–228
Brink AJ (1949) Coronary vessels in Bantu; preliminary report on coronary artery pattern in adult Bantu. Clin Proc 8:137–149
Brock JF, Bronte-Stewart B (1955) Arteriosclerosis in African populations. Minnesota Med 38:852–863
Bronte-Stewart B, Keys A, Brock JF (1955) Serum-cholesterol, diet and coronary heart disease. Lancer 2:1103–1107
Gillman T, Naidoo SS, Hathorn M (1957) Fat fibrinolysis and atherosclerosis in Africans. Lancet 2:696–697
Higginson J, Pepler WJ (1954) Fat intake, serum cholesterol concentration and atherosclrosis in the South African Bantu. II Atherosclerosis and coronary artery disease. J Clin Invest 33:1366–1371
Hutt MS, Coles R (1969) Postmortem findings in hypertensive subjects in Kampala Uganda. East Afr Med J 46:342–358
Isaacson C (1977) The changing pattern of heart disease in South African Blacks. S Afr Med J 52:793–798
Isaacson C (1978) Pathological changes in hypertension. S Afr Med J 53:994–995
Isaacson C, Kincaid-Smith P (1962) Study of the kidney in the Bantu with hypertension. Br Heart J 24:372–374
Jones JJ, Gelfand M, Kanengoni E (1974) Renin activity in Black hypertensive patients in Rhodesia. S Afr Med J 48:2223–2225
Kincaid-Smith P, McMichael J, Murphy EA (1958) The clinical course and pathology of hypertension with papilloedema (Malignant hypertension). Q J Med 27:117–153
Koate P, Couturier Y, Quenum C, Wade F (1971) Ischaemic cardiopathies in the African Negro as based on 16 cases of myocardial infarct and 5 cases of angina pectoris in the Senegalese at Dakar. Afr J Med Sci 2:207–216
Mersky C, Gordon H, Lackner H (1958) Diet, blood chemistry, blood coagulation and fibrinolysis in relation to coronary heart disease. An interracial study. S Afr Med J 32:855–856

Reef H, Isaacson C (1962) Atherosclerosis in the Bantu: The distribution of atheromatous lesions in Africans over 50 years of age. Circulation 25:66–72
Sacks MI (1960) Aortic and coronary atherosclerosis in the three racial groups in Cape Town. Circulation 22:96–109
Schrire V (1961) The comparative racial prevalence of ischaemic heart disease in Cape Town. Am J Cardiol 8:173–177
Schrire V, Uys CJ (1958) Cardiac infarction in the Bantu. Am J Cardiol 2:453–463
Schwartz MB, Schamroth L, Seftel HC (1958) The pattern of heart disease in the urbanized (Johannesburg) African. Med Proc 4:275–281
Seedat YK, Reddy J (1974) A study of 1000 South African Non White hypertensive patients. S Afr Med J 48:816–820
Seedat YK, Pillay N (1977) Myocardial infarction in the African hypertensive patient. Am Heart J 94:388–390
Seedat YK, Seedat MA, Nkomo MN (1978) The prevalence of hypertension in the Urban Zulu. S Afr Med J 53:923–927
Seftel HC (1973) Medicine and Society in South Africa – some plain speaking. Witwatersrand University Press, Johannesburg, p 14
Seftel HC (1978) The rarity of coronary heart disease in South African Blacks. S Afr Med J 54:99–105
Seftel HC, Kew MC (1970) Myocardial infarction in Johannesburg Bantu. S Afr Med J 44:8–13
Seftel HC, Schewitz LJ, Isaacson C (1960) Renal biopsy studies in hypertensive and renal disease in pregnancy. The Leech 30:128–133
Shaper AG (1972) Cardiovascular disease in the Tropics – III blood pressure and hypertension. Br Med J 3:805–807
Singer R (1959) Coronary arteries of the Bantu heart. S Afr Med J 33:467–468
Strong JP, Wainwright J, McGill HC (1959) Atherosclerosis in the Bantu. Circulation 20:1118–1127
Wainwright J (1961) Atheroma in the African (Bantu) in Natal. Lancet 1:366–368
Walker ARP (1969) Can expectation of life in Western populations be increased by changes in diet and manner of life? Part II. S Afr Med J 43:768–775
Walker ARP (1974) Atherosclerosis and nutrition with special reference to populations in Africa. S Afr Med J 48:481–484
Walker ARP (1975) The epidemiological emergence of ischaemic arterial diseases. Am Heart J 89:133–136
Walker ARP, Simson IW (1958) Mortality from cerebral vascular and coronary disease among the South African Bantu. Lancet 1:1126–1127
Williams AO (1969) Atherosclerosis in the Nigerian. J Pathol 99:219–235
Williams AO, Resch JA, Loewenson RB (1971) Comparative study on cerebral atherosclerosis between an African (Nigerian) and American population groups (Caucasian and Negroes). East Afr Med J 48:152–162
Wyndham CH (1979) Mortality from cardiovascular diseases in the various population groups in the Republic of South Africa. S Afr Med J 56:1023–1030

Chapter 3

Abrahams DG, Barton CJ, Cockshott WP, Edington GM, Weaver EJM (1962) Annular subvalvular left ventricular aneurysms. Q J Med 31:345–360
Baker LW, Houlder A (1973) Deep vein thrombosis in Bantu and Indian patients. S Afr Med J 47:1689–1692
Barlow JB, Bosman CK (1966) Aneurysmal protrusion of the posterior leaflet of the mitral valves. Am Heart J 71:166–178
Becker W, Schrire V (1969) Idiopathic mitral subannular left ventricular aneurysm in the Bantu. Am Heart J 78:28–33

Bittar N, Sosa JA (1968) The billowing mitral valve leaflet, report on fourteen patients. Circulation 38:763–770
Cardell BS, Hanley T (1951) Fatal case of giantcell or temporal arteritis. J Pathol Bact 63:587–597
Chesler E, Levin S, Du Plessis L, Freiman I, Rogers M, Joffe N (1966) The pattern of rheumatic heart disease in the urbanized Bantu of Johannesburg. S Afr Med J 40: 899–906
Cockshott WP, Antia A, Ikeme A, Uzodike VO (1967) Annular subvalvular aneurysms. Br J Radiol 40:424–435
Davis RH, Schuster B, Knoebel SB, Fisch C (1971) Myxomatous degeneration of the mitral valve. Am J Cardiol 28:449–455
Decker GAG, Samson ID, Schmaman A (1977) Abdominal aneurysm in South African Negroes due to intimomedial mucoid degeneration. Br J Surg 64:513–516
Drury RA, Mylius EA (1973) The changing pattern of pulmonary embolism in Ugandan Africans. Afr J Med Sci 5:369–381
Erdheim J (1930) Medionecrosis aortae idiopathica cystica. Virchows Arch Pathol Anat 276:187–229
Frable WJ (1969) Mucinous degeneration of the cardiac valves, the "floppy valve" syndrome. J Thorac Cardiovasc Surg 58:62–70
Gelfand M (1955) Giantcell arteritis with aneurysm formation in infant. Br Heart J 17:264–266
Gelfand M, Ross M (1976) Pulmonary embolism in the Rhodesian Black. S Afr Med J 50:19–21
Higginson J, Keeley KH (1951) An unusual cardiac aneurysm in a young adult. J Clin Pathol 4:342–349
Higginson J, Isaacson C, Simson I (1960) The pathology of cryptogenic heart disease. Arch Pathol 70:947–507
Isaacson C (1961) An idiopathic aortitis in young Africans. J Pathol Bact 81:69–79
Isaacson C (1977) The changing pattern of heart disease in South African Blacks. S Afr Med J 52:793–798
Isaacson C (1980) Myxomatous degeneration of the heart valves in Blacks. S Afr Med J 57:537–538
Isaacson C, Shnier M (1961) Aortitis: A review with a further case report of an idiopathic type in an African child. Med Proc 7:525–533
Isaacson C, Klachko DM, Wayburne S, Simson IW (1959) Aortitis in children. Lancet 2:542–544
Joffey SN (1974) Racial incidence of postoperative deep vein thrombosis in South Africa. Br J Surg 61:982–983
Kallichurum S (1969) Thrombo-embolic cor pulmonale in the Bantu in Durban. S Afr Med J 43:291–298
Lupi-Herrera E, Sánchez-Torres G, Marcushamer J, Mispireta J, Horwitz S, Vela JE (1977) Review. Takayasu's arteritis. Clinical study of 107 cases. Am Heart J 93: 94–103
Lurie AO (1960) Left ventricular aneurysm in the African. Br Heart J 22:181–188
Pepler WJ (1955) The incidence of degeneration of the aorta in South African Bantu. Part III. S Afr J Lab Clin Med 1:222–238
Pocock WA, Barlow JB (1971) An association between the billowing posterior mitral leaflet syndrome and congenital heart disease, particularly atrial septal defect. Am Heart J 81:720–722
Pomerance A (1969) Ballooning deformity (Mucoid degeneration) of atrioventricular valves. Br Heart J 31:343–351
Pomerance A, Davies MJ (1975) The pathology of the heart. Blackwell, Oxford
Robertson JH, Jackson JG (1960) Cardiac aneurysms in Nigeria. J Pathol Bact 80: 101–109

Schrire V (1958) The racial incidence of heart disease, Part II. Hypertension and valvular disease of the heart, Groote Schuur Hospital Cape Town. Am Heart J 56: 742–760

Schwartz MB, Schamroth L, Seftel HC (1958) The pattern of heart disease in the urbanized (Johannesburg) African. Med Proc 4:275–281

Seftel HC (1973) Medicine and society in South Africa – some plain speaking. Witwatersrand, Johannesburg, p 14

Seftel HC, Metz J, Lakier JB (1972) Cardiomyopathies in Johannesburg Bantu – I Aetiology and characteristics of beri-beri heart disease. S Afr Med J 46:1707–1713

Shaper AG (1972) Cardiovascular disease in the tropics – I Rheumatic heart. Br Med J 3:683–686

Shaper AG, Hutt MS, Coles RM (1968) Necropsy study of endomyocardial fibrosis and rheumatic heart disease in Uganda 1950–1965. Br Heart J 30:390–401

Spodick DH (1975) Rheumatic heart disease in South Africa. Br Med J 4:579

Ueno A, Awane Y, Wakabayachi A, Shimizu K (1967) Successfully operated obliterative brachiocephalic arteritis (Takayasu) associated with an elongated coarctation. Jpn Heart J 8:538–544

Walker ARP (1969) Can expectation of life in Western populations be increased by changes in diet and manner of life: Part II. S Afr Med J 43:768–775

Chapter 4

Astaldi G, Meardi G, Lisino T (1966) The iron content of jejunal mucosa obtained by Crosby's biopsy in hemochromatosis and hemosiderosis. Blood 28:70–82

Barnes HD (1945) A note on porphyrinuria with a resume of eleven South African cases. Clin Proc 4:269–279

Bolgert M, Cavinet J, Le Sourd M (1953) La porphyrie cutanée l'adulte; étude de neuf cas et description. Sem Hôp Paris 29:1587–1608

Bothwell TH, Bradlow BA (1960) Siderosis in the Bantu: A combined histopathological and chemical study. Arch Pathol 70:279–292

Bothwell TH, Isaacson C (1962) Siderosis in the Bantu: A comparison of incidence in males and females. Br Med J 1:522–524

Bothwell TH, van Doorn-Wittkampf HVW, du Preez ML, Alper T (1953) The absorption of iron: radioiron studies in idiopathic haemochromatosis, malnutritional cytosiderosis and transfusional haemosiderosis. J Lab Clin Med 41:836–848

Bothwell TH, Seftel H, Jacobs P, Torrance JD, Baumslag N (1964) Iron overload in Bantu subjects. Am J Clin Nutr 14:47–51

Bothwell TH, Abrahams C, Bradlow BA, Charlton RW (1965) Idiopathic and Bantu hemochromatosis. Arch Pathol 79:163–168

Bradlow B, Dunn J, Higginson J (1961) The effect of cirrhosis on iron storage. Am J Pathol 39:221–235

Buchanan WM (1969a) Aetiology of extrahepatic epithelial iron deposits in siderosis in Bantu. J Clin Pathol 22:296–300

Buchanan WM (1969b) The role of collateral circulation in the production of epithelial iron deposits in Africans with siderosis and cirrhosis. S Afr J Med Sci 34:29–34

Buchanan WM (1970) Peritonitis and Bantu siderosis. S Afr Med J 44:43–44

Buchanan WM (1971) Shock in Bantu siderosis. Am J Clin Pathol 55:401–406

Buchanan WM (1972) Iron overload. Centr Afr J Med 18:35–40

Campbell JAH (1963–64) Pathological aspects of hexachlorobenzene feeding in rats. S Afr J Lab Clin Med 9–10:203–211

Charlton RW, Jacobs P, Seftel H (1964) Effect of alcohol on iron absorption. Br Med J 2:1427–1429

Charlton RW, Bothwell TH, Mayet FGH, Simson IW (1971) Liver iron stores in different population groups in South Africa. S Afr Med J 45:524–529

Conrad ME Jr, Berman A, Brosby WH (1962) Iron kinetics in Laennec's cirrhosis. Gastroenterology 43:385–390
Davies G, Dymock I, Harry J, Williams R (1972) Deposition of melanin and iron in ocular structures in haemochromatosis. Br J Ophthalmol 56:338–342
Davis AE, Badenoch J (1962) Iron absorption in pancreatic disease. Lancet 2:6–8
Epstein JH, Pinsky JB (1965) Porphyria cutanea tarda. Arch Dermatol 92:362–366
Epstein JH, Redeker AG (1968) Porphyria cutanea tarda. A study of the effect of phlebotomy. New Engl. J Med 279:1301–1304
Felsher BF, Redeker AG (1972) The relationship of iron to hepatic uroporphyrin synthesis in porphyria cutanea tarda. Clin Res 20:182
Forbes JI (1966) Tightness of the skin over the feet and lower limb associated with haemosiderosis. S Afr Med J 40:656–660
Galambos JT (1975) Hemochromatosis. Am J Gastroenterol 64:169–174
Gelfand M (1955) Pophyria in the Rhodesian African. Centr Afr J Med 1:281–285
Gillman J, Gillman T (1945) Structure of the liver in pellagra. Arch Pathol 40:239–263
Gillman J, Gillman T (1951) Perspectives in human nutrition. Grune & Stratton, New York
Gillman J, Mandelstam J, Gillman T (1945) A comparison of chemical and histological estimations of the iron and copper content of the livers of Africans in relation to the pathogenesis of cytosiderosis and cirrhosis (haemochromatosis). S Afr J Med Sci 10:109–136
Gillman J, Gillman T, Mandelstam J, Gilbert C (1947) Cytosiderosis and genesis of arteriosclerosis and other fibrous tissue reactions. Nature 159:875–876
Gillman T, Lamont NM , Hathorn M (1957) Haemochromatosis, African nutritional siderosis, and experimental siderosis in animals. Lancet 2:173–175
Gillman T, Hathorn M, Lamont NM (1958) Liver disease in Durban Africans. S Afr J Med Sci 23:187–200
Gillman T, Hathorn M, Canham PAS (1959) Experimental dietary siderosis. Am J Pathol 35:349–367
Golberg L, Smith JP (1960) Iron overloading and hepatic vulnerability. Am J Pathol 36:125–145
Grusin H, Samuel E (1957) A syndrome of osteoporosis in Africans and its relationship to scurvy. Am J Clin Nutr 5:644–650
Hartley WJ, Mullins J, Lawson BM (1959) Nutritional siderosis in the bovine. N Z Vet J 7:99–105
Hegsted DM, Finch CA, Kinney TD (1949) Influence of diet on iron absorption, interrelation of iron and phosphorus. J Exp Med 90:147–156
Higginson J, Gerritsen TH, Walker ARP (1953) Siderosis in the Bantu of Southern Africa. Am J Pathol 29:779–815
Higginson J, Grobbelaar BG, Walker ARP (1957) Hepatic fibrosis and cirrhosis in man in relation to malnutrition. Am J Pathol 33:29–53
Höjer JA (1923) Scurvy. Acta Paediatr Scand (Suppl) 3:8–278
Isaacson C, Seftel HC, Keeley KJ, Bothwell TH (1961) Siderosis in the Bantu: The relationship between iron overload and cirrhosis. J Lab Clin Med 58:845–853
Jones NL (1962) Irreversible shock in haemochromatosis. Lancet 1:569–572
Keeley KJ (1963/64) The relationship between diabetes and porphyria. S Afr J Lab Clin Med 9/10:304
Keeley KJ, Bothwell TH, Kramer S (1960) High plasma-iron in porphyria. Lancet 1:601
Kinney TD, Hegsted DM, Finch CA (1949) Influence of diet on iron absorption: Pathology of iron excess. J Exp Med 90:137–145
Kinney TD, Finch CA, Kaufman N, Hegsted M, Partington PF (1950) The relationship of the pancreas to the absorption of iron. Am J Pathol 26:746
Kinney TD, Kaufman N, Klavins J (1955) Effect of ethionine-induced pancreatic damage on iron absorption. J Exp Med 102:151–156

Kramer S (1963) Iron metabolism in the porphyrias. S Afr J Lab Clin Med 9:283–287
Kushner JP, Lee GR, Nacht S (1972) The role of iron in the pathogenesis of porphyria cutanea tarda. J Clin Invest 51:3044–3051
Lamont N McE, Hathorn M (1960) Increased plasma iron and liver pathology in Africans with porphyria. S Afr Med J 34:279–281
Lamont N McE, Hathorn M, Joubert SM (1961) Porphyria in the African. A study of 100 cases. Q J Med 30:373–392
Lynch SR, Berelowitz I, Seftel HC (1967) Osteoporosis in Johannesburg Bantu males: Its relationship to siderosis and ascorbic acid deficiency. Am J Clin Nutr 20:799–807
Lynch SR, Seftel HC, Torrance JD (1967) Accelerated oxidative catabolism of ascorbic acid in siderotic Bantu. Am J Clin Nutr 20:641–647
Lynch SR, Seftel HC, Wapnick AA, Charlton RW, Bothwell TH (1970) Some aspects of calcium metabolism in normal and osteoporotic Bantu subjects with special reference to the effects of iron overload and ascorbic acid depletion. S Afr J Med Sci 35:45–56
MacDonald RA (1963) Wine and iron in haemochromatosis. Lancet 1:727
MacDonald RA, Jones RS, Pechet GS (1965) Folic acid deficiency and hemochromatosis. Arch Pathol 80:153–160
MacPhail AP, Simon MO, Torrance JD, Bothwell TH, Isaacson C (1979) Changing patterns of dietary iron overload in Black South Africans. Am J Clin Nutr 32:1272–1278
Martin CM, Handl JH, Finland M (1963) Enhancement of acute bacterial infections in rats and mice by iron and their inhibition by human transferrin. J Infect Dis 112: 158–163
Mazur A, Sackler M (1967) Haemochromatosis and hepatic xanthine oxidase. Lancet 1:254–255
Mirvish SS (1975) Blocking of the formation of N-nitrose compounds with ascorbic acid in vitro and in vivo. Ann NY Acad Sci 258:175–180
Murray MJ, Murray A, Murray CJ (1980) The salutary effect of milk on amoebiasis and its reversal by iron. Br Med J 280:1351–1352
Rather LJ (1956) Hemochromatosis and hemosiderosis: Does iron overload cause diffuse fibrosis of the liver? Am J Med 21:857–866
Schwartz SO (1956) Exogenous hemochromatosis: Concept and general description. Am J Clin Pathol 26:744–749
Schultz EJ, Swanepoel H (1962) Scorbutic pseudoscleroderma: An aspect of Bantu siderosis. S Afr Med J 36:367–372
Seftel HC, Isaacson C, Bothwell TH (1960) The relationship between siderosis and diabetes in the Bantu. S Afr J Med Sci 25:89–98
Seftel HC, Keeley KJ, Isaacson C, Bothwell TH (1961) Siderosis in the Bantu: The clinical incidence of haemochromatosis in diabetic subjects. J Lab Clin Med 58: 837–844
Seftel HC, Abrams GJ, Charlton RW, Abrahams C, Rubenstein A, Jacobs P, Bothwell TH (1963) Osteoporosis and siderosis in Africans. S Afr J Med Sci 28:115
Seftel HC, Charlton RW, Jacobs P, Bothwell TH (1964) Osteoporosis, scurvy and siderosis in South African Bantu. S Afr J Med Sci 29:97
Seftel HC, Malkin C, Schmaman A, Abrahams C, Lynch SR, Charlton RW, Bothwell TH (1966) Osteoporosis, scurvy and siderosis in Johannesburg Bantu. Br Med J 1: 642–646
Shaper AG (1958) Porphyria in Africa. Centr Afr J Med 4:411–420
Strachan AS (1929) Haemosiderosis and haemochromatosis in South African natives, with comment on the aetiology of haemochromatosis. M.D. Thesis, University of Glasgow
Taljaard JJD, Shanley BC, Deppe WM, Joubert SM (1972) Porphyrin metabolism in experimental hepatic sidersosis in the rat. Br J Haematol 23:513–519

Taylor J, Stiven D, Reid EW (1931) Haemochromatosis in a depancreatised cat. J Pathol Bact 34:793–797

Taylor J, Stiven D, Reid EW (1935) Experimental and idiopathic siderosis in cats. J Pathol Bact 41:397–404

Torrance JD, Bothwell TH (1968) A simple technique for measuring storage iron concentrations in formalinised liver samples. S Afr J Med Sci 33:9–11

Uys CJ, Eales L (1963) The histopathology of the liver in acquired (symptomatic) porphyria. S Afr J Lab Clin Med 9:190–197

Wainwright J (1957) Siderosis in the African. S Afr J Lab Clin Med 3:1–28

Walker ARP, Arvidsson UB (1950) Iron intake and haemochromatosis in the Bantu. Nature 166:438–439

Walker ARP, Arvidsson UB (1953) Iron overload in the South African Bantu. Trans R Soc Trop Med Hyg 47:536–548

Walker ARP, Strydom ESP, Reynolds PA (1955) The composition and density of thoracic vertebral bodies from South African Bantu adults habituated to a very high iron intake. S Afr J Lab Clin Med 1:254–262

Wapnick AA, Lynch SR, Krawitz P, Seftel HC, Charlton RW, Bothwell TH (1968) Effects of iron overload on ascorbic acid metabolism. Br Med J 3:704–707

Wapnick AA, Bothwell TH, Seftel HC (1970) The relationship between serum iron levels and ascorbic acid stores in siderotic Bantu. Br J Haematol 19:271–276

Wapnick AA, Lynch SR, Seftel HC, Charlton RW, Bothwell TH (1971) The effect of siderosis and ascorbic acid depletion on bone metabolism, with special reference to osteoporosis in the Bantu. Br J Nutr 25:367–376

Chapter 5

Anthony PP (1972) Primary carcinoma of the liver. A study of 282 cases in Ugandan Africans. J Pathol 110:37–48

Back E, Bras G (1958) Follow-up of cases of kwashiorkor. W Indian Med J 7:160

Bagshawe AF, Gacengi DM, Cameron CH, Dorman J, Dane DS (1975) Hepatitis B antigen and liver cancer – a population based study in Kenya. Br J Cancer 31:581–584

Becker BJP (1957) The liver in haemochromatosis. Lancet 2:598–599

Berry DM, Bras G (1957) Venous occlusion of the liver in crotalaria and senecio poisoning. N Am Vet 38:323–328

Bersohn I, Macnab GM, Pyzikowska J, Kew MC (1974) The prevalence of hepatitis B (Australia) antigen in South Africa. S Afr Med J 48:941–942

Bothwell TH, Bradlow BA (1960) Siderosis in the Bantu: A combined histopatholog-i-cal and chemical study. Arch Pathol 70:279–292

Bothwell TH, Isaacson C (1962) Siderosis in the Bantu: A comparison of incidence in males and females. Br Med J 1:522–524

Bradshaw E, Harington JS (1976) Temporal changes in primary liver cancer in Black goldminers from Mozambique. S Afr Med J 50:2022

Brock JF (1954) Survey of world situation on kwashiorkor. Ann NY Acad Sci 57: 696–713

Butler WH (1964) Acute toxicity of aflatoxin BI in rats. Br J Cancer 18:756–762

Christoffersen P, Eghöje K, Huhl E (1973) Mallory bodies in liver biopsies from chronic alcoholics. A comparative morphological, biochemical and clinical study of two groups of chronic alcoholics with and without Mallory bodies. Scand J Gastroenterol 8:341–346

Gillman J, Gillman T (1945) Structure of the liver in pellagra. Arch Pathol 40:239–263

Gillman J, Gillman T (1951) Perspectives in human nutrition. Grune & Stratton, New York

Gillman T, Hathorn M, Lamont NM (1958) Liver disease in Durban Africans. S Afr J Med Sci 23;187–200

Grusin H (1955) Potassium dichromate as a witchdoctor's remedy: Five cases of poisoning. S Afr Med J 29:117–120
Harington JS, McGlashan ND, Bradshaw E, Geddes EW, Purves LR (1975) A spatial and temporal analysis of four cancers in African gold miners from Southern Africa. Br J Cancer 31:665–678
Higginson J (1955) Relation of carcinoma of the liver to cirrhosis, malaria, syphilis and parasitic diseases. Schweiz Z Pathol Bakt 18:625–643
Higginson J, Gerritsen TH, Walker ARP (1953) Siderosis in the Bantu of Southern Africa. Am J Pathol 29:779–815
Higginson J, Grobbelaar BG, Walker ARP (1957) Hepatic fibrosis and cirrhosis in man in relation to malnutrition. Am J Pathol 33:29–45
Hill KR, Stephenson CF, Filshie I (1958) Hepatic veno-occlusive disease produced experimentally in rats by the injection of monocrotaline. Lancet 1:623
Isaacson C (1966) The aetiology of cirrhosis and hepatoma in the Bantu – an appraisal. S Afr Med J 40:11–13
Isaacson C (1978) The changing pattern of liver disease in South African Blacks. S Afr Med J 53:365–368
Isaacson C, Seftel HC, Keeley KJ, Bothwell TH (1961) Siderosis in the Bantu. The relationship between iron overload and cirrhosis. J Lab Clin Med 58:845–853
Jelliffe DB, Bras G, Mukherjee KL (1957) Venolocclusive disease of the liver and Indian childhood cirrhosis. Arch Dis Child 32:369–385
Kew MC, Miller GB, Stevenson CM, Macnab DM, Bersohn I (1974) The prevalence of virus B hepatitis in South African Blacks. S Afr Med J 48:1837–1838
Lee FI (1966) Cirrhosis and hepatoma in alcoholics. Gut 7:77–85
Macnab GM, Urbanowicz JM, Geddes EW, Kew MC (1976) Hepatitis-B surface antigen and antibody in Bantu patients with primary hepatocellular cancer. Br J Cancer 33: 544–548
Maynard EP, Sadikali F, Anthony PP, Barker LF (1970) Hepatitis-associated antigen and cirrhosis in Uganda. Lancet 2:1326–1328
MacPhail AP, Simon MO, Torrance JD, Bothwell TH, Isaacson C (1979) Changing patterns of dietary iron overload in Black South Africans. Am J Clin Nutr 32:1272–1278
Neame PB, Pillay BKG (1964) Spontaneous hypoglycaemia, hepatic and renal necrosis following intake of herbal medicines. S Afr Med J 38:729–732
Oettle AG (1965) The aetiology of primary carcinoma of the liver in Africa: A critical appraisal of previous ideas with an outline of the mycotoxin hypothesis. S Afr Med J 39:817–825
Peers FG, Linsell GA (1973) Dietary aflatoxins and liver cancer: A population based study in Kenya. Br J Cancer 27:473–484
Primack A, Vogel CL, Barker LF (1973) Immunological studies in Uganda patients with hepatocellular carcinoma. Br Med J 1:16–19
Rhodes K (1957) Two types of liver disease in Jamaican children. W Ind Med J 6:73–93
Seftel HC, Isaacson C, Bothwell TH (1960) The relationship between siderosis and diabetes in the Bantu. S Afr J Med Sci 25:89–98
Selzer G, Parker RGF (1951) Senecio poisoning exhibiting as Chiari's syndrome: A report on twelve cases. Am J Pathol 27:885–907
Sherlock S, Fox RA, Niazi SP, Scheuer PJ (1970) Chronic liver disease and primary liver-cell cancer with hepatitis-associated antigen in serum (Australia). Lancet 1: 1243–1247
Stein H (1957) Veno-occlusive disease of the liver in African children. Br Med J 1: 1496–1499
Stein H, Isaacson C (1960) Cirrhosis of the liver in childhood: Its relationship to protein malnutrition (kwashiorkor). Med Proc 6:7–13
Stein H, Isaacson C (1962) Veno-occlusive disease of the liver. Br Med J 1:372–374

Steiner PE (1960) Cancer of the liver and cirrhosis in Trans-Saharan Africa and the United States of America. Cancer 13:1085–1166

Theodorpopulos G, Archimandritis A, Angelopoulos B (1975) Letter: Australia antigen and malignant hepatoma. Ann Intern Med 82:809–810

Tong MJ, Sun SC, Schaeffer BT, Chang NK, Lo KJ, Peters RL (1971) Hepatitis-associated antigen and hepatocellular carcinoma in Taiwan. Ann Intern Med 75:687–691

Torres FO, Purchase IFH, Van der Watt JJ (1970) The aetiology of primary liver cancer in the Bantu. J Pathol 102:163–169

Trowell HC, Davies JNP, Dean RFA (1954) Kwashiorkor. Arnold, London

Van Rensburg SJ, Van der Watt JJ, Purchase IFH, Coutinho LP, Markham R (1974) Primary liver cancer rate and aflatoxin intake in a high cancer area. S Afr Med J 48: 2508A–2508D

Vogel CL, Anthony PP, Mody N, Barker LF (1970) Hepatitis-associated antigen in Ugandan patients with hepatocellular carcinoma. Lancet 2:621–624

Wainwright (1957) Siderosis in the African. S Afr J Lab Clin Med 3:1–28

Wainwright J, Schonland MM (1977) Toxic hepatitis in Black patients in Natal. S Afr Med J 51:571–573

Waterlow JC (1948) Spec Rep Med Res Counc No 263. London

Chapter 6

Anand SV, Davey WW, Cohen B (1967) Tumours of the jaw in West Africa: A review of 256 patients. Br J Surg 54:901–917

Anthony PP, Vogel CL, Sakikali F, Barker LF, Peterson MR (1972) Hepatitis-associated antigen and antibody in Uganda: Correlation of serological testing with histopathology. Br Med J 1:403–406

Beardmore GL (1972) Melanoma and skin cancer. In: McCarthy WW (ed) Proceedings of the International Cancer Conference held in Sydney 13th–17th March 1972. Government Printer, Sidney, pp 39–64

Bhoola KD, Bhamjee A (1976) A comparative study of ovarian tumours in Black and Indian patients. S Afr Med J 50:1935–1936

Boyland E, Walker SA (1975) Thiocyanate catalysis of nitrosamine formation and some dietary implications. In: Bogorski P, Walker EA (eds) N-nitroso compounds in the environment. IARC Scientific Publications No 9. International Agency for Research on Cancer, Lyon, p 132

Bradshaw E, Harington JS (1976) Temporal changes in primary liver cancer in Black goldminers from Mozambique. S Afr Med J 50:2022

Bremner CG, Ackerman LV (1970) Polyps and carcinoma of the large bowel in the South African Bantu. Cancer 26:991–999

Burkitt DP (1969) Related disease – related cause? Lancet 2:1229–1231

Burkitt DP (1971) Some lessons from cancer patterns in Africa. Med Proc 17:70–74

Burrell JW, Roach WA, Shadwell A (1966) Oesophageal cancer in the Bantu of Transkei associated with mineral deficiency in garden plants. J Natl Cancer Inst 36:201–209

Chabon AB, Takeuchi S, Sommers SC (1974) Histologic differences in breast carcinoma of Japanese and American women. Cancer 33:1577–1579

Charlewood GP, Frylinck R (1951) Some discrepancies in disease incidence between the European and the South African Negro (Bantu). S Afr Med J 25:569–574

Correa P, O'Conor GT (1971) Epidemiologic patterns of Hodgkin's disease. Int J Cancer 8:192–201

Crespi M, Grassi A, Amiri G, Munoz N, Aramesh B, Mojtabai A, Casale V (1979) Oesophageal lesions in Northern Iran: A premalignant condition. Lancet 2:217–220

Cuello C, Correa P, Eisenberg H (1969) Geographic pathology of thyroid carcinoma. Cancer 23:230–239

Davey WW (1964) Renal tumours in Nigeria. Br J Urol 36:340–346
Davies AGM, Davies JNP (1960) Tumours of the jaw in Uganda Africans. Acta Un Int Cancer 16:1320–1324
Davies JNP (1957) Cancer in relation to other disease in Africa. Acta Un Int Cancer 13:898–903
Davies JNP (1962) Kaposi's sarcoma: A re-evaluation based on the disease in Africans. Acta Un Int Cancer 18:330–363
Davies JNP (1970) Epidemiology of breast cancer (Letter to the Editor). Int J Cancer 5:157
Davies JNP, Dodge OG, Burkitt DP (1964) Salivary-gland tumours in Uganda. Cancer 17:1310–1322
Davies JNP, Knowelden J, Wilson BA (1965) Incidence rates of cancer in Kyadondo County, Uganda, 1954–1960. J Natl Cancer Inst 35:789–821
Davies JNP, Tank R, Meyer R, Thurston P (1968) Cancer of the integumentary tissues in Uganda Africans: The basis for prevention. J Natl Cancer Inst 41:31–51
Decker GAG (1974) Carcinoma of the thyroid at Baragwanath Hospital. S Afr J Surg 12:155–158
De Moor GW, Berry AV (1976) Cancer of the cervix: Factors of significance in the prognosis. S Afr Cancer Bull 20:152–158
Dixon FJ, Moore RA (1953) Testicular tumours: clinicopathological study. Cancer 6: 427–454
Dodge OG (1962) Tumours of the bladder in Uganda Africans. Acta Un Int Cancer 18: 548–552
Dodge OG (1965) Carcinoma of the penis in East Africans. Br J Urol 37:223–226
Dodge OG (1965) Tumours of the jaw, odontogenic tissues and maxillary antrum (excluding Burkitt Lymphoma) in Uganda Africans. Cancer 18:205–215
Doll R (1975) The epidemiology of cancers of the breast and reproductive system. Scot Med J 20:305–315
Editorial (1973) Nephroblastoma: an index reference cancer. Lancet 2:651
Editorial (1974) Leads in oesophageal cancer. Lancet 2:504
Fisher ER, Gregoria R, Redmond C, Vellios F, Sommers SC, Fisher B (1975) Pathologic findings from the national surgical adjuvant breast project. Cancer 35:247–253
Freedman RS, Joosting ACC, Ryan JT, Nkosi S (1974) A study of associated factors, including genital herpes, in Black women with cervical carcinoma in Johannesburg. S Afr Med J 48:1748–1752
Fripp PH (1965) Bilharziasis and bladder cancer. Br J Cancer 19:292–296
Froman C, Lipschitz R (1970) Demography of tumours of the central nervous system among the Bantu (African) population of the Transvaal, South Africa. J Neurosurg 32:660–664
Giraud RMA, Rippey R, Rippey JJ (1975) Malignant melanoma of the skin in Black Africans. S Afr Med J 49:665–668
Gresh S, Lewis MG (1967) Ovarian tumours in Ugandan Africans. East Afr Med J 44: 487–492
Gunderson LL, Weems WS, Hebertson RM, Plenk HP (1974) Correlation of histopathology with clinical results following radiation therapy for carcinoma of the cervix. Am J Roentgenol 120:74–87
Harington JS (1975) Epidemiology and aetiology of cancer of the uterine cervix – including the detection of carcinogenic N-Nitrosamines in the human vault. S Afr Med J 49:443–445
Higginson J (1968) Distribution of different patterns of cancer. Israel J Med Sci 4: 457–468
Higginson J, Oettle AG (1960) Cancer incidence in the Bantu and "Cape Coloured" races of South Africa: Report of a cancer survey in the Transvaal (1953–1955). J Natl Cancer Inst 24:589–671

Hill MJ, Goddard P, Williams REO (1971) Gut bacteria and aetiology of cancer of the breast. Lancet 2:472–473

Hinder RA, Schmaman A (1969) Bilharziasis and squamous carcinoma of the bladder. S Afr Med J 43:617–618

Isaacson C, Selzer G, Kaye V, Greenberg M, Woodruff JD, Davies J, Ninin D, Vetten D, Andrews M (1978) Cancer in the urban Blacks of South Africa. S Afr Cancer Bull 22:49–84

Ivankovic S, Preusemann R, Schmähl D, Zeller IW (1975) Prevention by ascorbic acid of in vivo formation of N-nitroso compounds. In: Bogorski P, Walker EA (eds) N-nitroso compounds in the environment. IARC Scientific Publications No 9. International Agency for Research on Cancer, Lyon, p 101

Junaid TA, Hendrickse JPdeV, Oladiran B (1974) Choriocarcinoma in Ibadan Nigeria: Epidemiological aspects. J Natl Cancer Inst 53:1597–1599

Kariyabwire WM, Lewis MG, Ziegler JL, Loefler I (1968) Malignant melanoma in Uganda. East Afr Med J 45:498–507

Keen P, De Moor NG, Shapiro MP, Cohen L (1955) The aetiology of respiratory tract cancer in the South African Bantu. Br J Cancer 9:528–538

Kew MC, Geddes EW, Macnab GM, Bersohn I (1974) Hepatitis – B antigen and cirrhosis in Bantu patients with primary liver cancer. Cancer 34:539–541

Lauren P (1965) The two histological main types of gastric carcinoma. Diffuse and so-called intestinal-type carcinoma. Acta Pathol Microbiol Scand 64:31–49

Linsell CA, Martyn R (1962) The Kenya cancer registry. East Afr Med J 39:642–648

Louis S, Keet PC (1964) A survey of supratentorial gliomas and meningiomas. S Afr Med J 38:949–953

Lukes RJ, Cryver LF, Hall TC, Rappaport H, Ruben P (1966) Report of the nomenclature committee. Cancer Res 26:1311

Marasas WFO, Van Rensburg SJ, Mirocha CJ (1979) Incidence of fusarium species and the mycotoxins deoxynivalenol and zearalenone in corn produced in eosophageal cancer areas in Transkei. Agricultural and Food Chemistry 27:1108–1112

McGlashan ND, Walters CL (1969) Nitrosamines in South African alcoholic drinks in relation to oesophageal cancer. S Afr Med J 43:800

McGlashan ND, Walters CL, McLean AEM (1968) Nitrosamines in African alcoholic spirits and oesophageal cancer. Lancet 2:1017

McIllmurray MB, Langman MJS (1975) Progress report – Large bowel cancer: Causation and management. Gut 17:815–820

Mingxin L, Shixin L, Chuan J, Mingyao W, Shujun C, Changlian J (1979) Formation of carcinogenic N-nitroso compounds in corn-bread inoculated with fungi. Scientia Sinica 22:471–477

Morrow RH, Sai FT, Barker LF (1971) Australia antigen and hepatitis in Accra, Ghana. Br Med J 4:389–390

Morson BC (1969) Pathology of the gastrointestinal tract. Springer, Berlin Heidelberg New York

Mosadomi A (1975) Odontogenic tumours in an African population: Analysis of 29 cases seen over a 5 year period. Oral Surg 40:502–521

Movsas S (1966) Prostatic obstruction in the African and Asiatic. Br J Surg 53:538–543

Munoz N, Correa P, Cuello C, Duque E (1968) Histologic types of gastric carcinoma in high and low risk areas. Int J Cancer 3:809–818

Ng ABP, Atkins NB (1973) Histological cell type and DNA value in the prognosis of squamous cell cancer of uterine cervix. Br J Cancer 28:323–331

Nochomovitz LE, Kahn LB (1974) Tyrosine crystals in pleomorphic adenomas of the salivary gland. Arch Pathol 97:141–142

Oettle AG (1962) Geographical and racial differences in the frequency of Kaposi's sarcoma as evidence of environmental or genetic causes. Acta Un Int Cancer 18: 330–363

Oettle AG (1963) Skin cancer in Africa. Natl Cancer Inst Monogr 10–11:197–214
Oettle AG (1963) Regional variations in the frequency of Bantu oesophageal cancer cases admitted to hospital in South Africa. S Afr Med J 37:434–439
Oettle AG (1964) Cancer in Africa, especially in regions south of the Sahara. J Natl Cancer Inst 33:383–436
Oettle AG (1965) Aetiology of primary carcinoma of the liver in Africa: a critical appraisal of previous ideas with an outline of the mycotoxin hypothesis. S Afr Med J 39:817–825
Olisa EG, Kovi J, Kennedy J, Kish MH, Lanava TS, Williams AO (1977) Hodgkin's disease in American Negroes: Histological classification of the disease in 143 untreated patients and age distribution. Am J Clin Pathol 66:537–544
Park WW (1971) Chorio-carcinoma, a study of its pathology. Heinemann, London
Pearson JB (1963) Carcinoma of the breast in Nigeria – A study of 100 patients. Br J Cancer 17:559–565
Prates MD, Gillman J (1959) Carcinoma of the urinary bladder in the Portuguese East African with special reference to bilharzial cystitis and preneoplastic reactions. S Afr J Med Sci 24:13–40
Proctor NSF (1955) Intracranial tumours and cysts in the South African Bantu. Proc 2nd Int Congr Neuropathol, London, pp 99–103
Reagan JW (1974) Cellular pathology and uterine cancer. Am J Clin Pathol 62:150–164
Rippey JJ, Schmaman A (1972) Essays on tropical dermatology. Excerpta Medica (Amsterdam) 2:98–115
Roche WD, Norris HJ (1975) Microinvasive carcinoma of the cervix. Cancer 36:180–186
Rubio CA, Söderberg G, Einhorn N (1974) Histological and follow-up studies in cases of micro-invasive carcinoma of the uterine cervix. Acta Pathol Microbiol Scand (A) 82:397–410
Schmaman A, Smith I, Ackerman LV (1970) Benign fibro-osseous lesions of the mandible and maxilla: A review of 35 cases. Cancer 26:303–312
Schoental R, Joffe AZ (1974) Lesions induced in rodents by extracts from cultures of Fusarium poae and F. sporotrichioides. J Pathol 112:37–42
Schonland M, Bradshaw E (1968) Cancer in the Natal African and Indian 1964–1966. Int J Cancer 3:304–316
Schonland M, Bradshaw E (1968) Cancer in the Natal African 1964–1966 – cancer morbidity incidence and geographical pathology in Natal Hinterland. S Afr J Med Sci 33:33–42
Schonland M, Bradshaw E (1969) Oesophageal cancer in Natal Bantu: A review of 516 cases. S Afr Med J 43:1028–1031
Schonland M, Bradshaw E (1969) Cancer of the lung in Natal Bantu – a new cancer problem: A review of 472 cases 1964–66. S Afr Med J 43:1958–1960
Shear M (1977) Paper presented at Fifty-fifth Annual Meeting of the International Association for Dental Research, March 31–April 3
Slavin G, Cameron HMacD (1969) Ameloblastomas in Africans from Tanzania and Uganda. Br J Cancer 23:31–38
Te Groen LHT, Rose EF (1974) A preliminary investigation into the incidence of cancer of the cervix. S Afr Med J 48:2341–2345
Templeton AC (1973) Tumours in a tropical country: A survey of Uganda 1964–68. Heinemann, London
Torres FO, Purchase IFH, Van der Watt JJ (1970) The aetiology of primary liver cancer in the Bantu. J Pathol 102:163–169
Uys CJ (1956) Tumours of the kidney in Bantu races of South Africa; pathological study based on 3707 consecutive autopsies. Br J Urol 28:75–88
Van Rensburg SJ, Kirsipuu A, Coutinho LP, Van der Watt JJ (1975) Circumstances associated with the contamination of food by aflatoxin in a high primary liver cancer area. S Afr Med J 49:877–883

Vianna NJ, Thind IS, Louria DB, Polan A, Firmiss V, Davies JNP (1977) Epidemiologic and histologic patterns of Hodgkin's disease in Blacks. Cancer 40:3133–3139
Vogel CL, Anthony PP, Mody N, Barker LF (1970) Hepatitis-associated antigen in Ugandan patients with hepatocellular carcinoma. Lancet 2:621–624
Wainwright J, Roach GG (1957) Malignant neoplastic disease in Europeans, Africans and Indians in Natal. S Afr Cancer Bull 1:162–170
Walker ARP (1971) Diet, bowel motility, faeces composition and colonic cancer. S Afr Med J 45:377–379
Winship T (1958) Malignant tumours of the thyroid gland. In: Raven RW (ed) Cancer, vol 2. Butterworth, London
Wright CJ (1967) Thyrotoxicosis in the African, report of eight cases. East Afr Med J 44:455–463
Wynder EL, Kmet J, Dungal N, Segi M (1963) An epidemiological investigation of gastric cancer. Cancer 16:1461–1496

Chapter 7

Bureau Y, Barriere H (1958) Ulcerating and mutilating trophic lesions of the lower limbs. Br J Dermatol 70:372–377
Factor SM (1976) Intramyocardial small-vessel disease in chronic alcoholism. Am Heart J 92:561–575
Fagerberg SE (1959) Diabetic neuropathy; a clinical and histological study on the significance of vascular affections. Acta Med Scand 164 Suppl 345:1–97
Isaacson C (1977) Idiopathic neurotrophic feet in Blacks. A pathological study. S Afr Med J 52:845–848
Perdikis P, Bremner C (1969) Idiopathic neurotrophic feet in Bantu patients. S Afr J Surg 7:171–178
Pintar K, Wolansky BM, Gubbay ER (1965) Alcoholic cardiomyopathy. Canad Med Assoc J 93:103–107
Trope GE, Crookes RC (1975) Idiopathic neurotrophic feet in Blacks. S Afr Med J 49: 2157–2160

Chapter 8

Higginson J, Isaacson C, Simson I (1960) The pathology of cryptogenic heart disease. Arch Pathol 70:497–507
Olson LC, Bourgeois CG Jr, Cotton RB, Harikul S, Grossman RA, Smith TJ (1971) Encephalopathy and fatty degeneration of the viscera in north eastern Thailand. Clinical syndrome and epidemiology. Paediatr 47:707–716
Seftel HC (1973) Cardiomyopathies in Johannesburg Bantu. S Afr Med J 47:321–324
Shnier MH, Isaacson C (1965) Perinatal mortality in the Bantu. S Afr Med J 39:676–679
Smythe PM, Swanepoel A, Campbell JAH (1962) The heart in kwashiorkor. Br Med J 1:67–73
Stein H, Ellis US (1974) The low birthweight African baby. Arch Dis Child 49:156–159
Stein H, Isaacson C (1960) Cirrhosis of the liver in childhood, its relationship to protein malnutrition (Kwashiorkor). Med Proc 6:7–13
Stein H, Mouton SCE (1979) Neonatal mortality in a Black urban community. S Afr Med J 55:413–415
Trowell HC, Davies JNP, Dean RFA (1954) Kwashiorkor. Arnold, London
Van Rensburg SJ, Kirsipuu A, Pereira Coutinho L, Van der Watt JJ (1975) Circumstances associated with the contamination of food by aflatoxin in a high primary liver cancer area. S Afr Med J 49:877–883
Wharton BA, Balmer SE, Somers K, Templeton AC (1969) The myocardium in kwashiorkor. Q J Med 38:107–116

I would like to thank the editors of these journals for permission to quote extensively from articles and to reproduce the photographs and charts listed.

Arch Dis Child 39:610–617 (1964) Cardiomyopathy in African children. Stein H, Shnier H, Waburne S, Isaacson C: Figure 3

Arch Pathol 70:497–507 (1960) The pathology of cryptogenic heart disease. Higginson J, Isaacson C, Simson I

S Afr Med J 52:793–798 (1977) Changing patterns of heart disease in South African Blacks. Isaacson C: Tables 2 and 3

Lancet 2:542–546 (1959) Aortitis in children. Isaacson C, Klachko DN, Wayburne S, Simson IW: Figures I and II

J Pathol Bacteriol 81:69–79 (1961) An idiopathic aortitis in young Africans. Isaacson C: Figure 5

Br J Surg 64:513–516 (1977) Abdominal aneurysms in South African Negroes due to intimomedial mucoid degeneration. Decker GAG, Samson ID, Schmaman A: Figures 1, 2, 3, and 4

Br Med J 1:522–524 (1962) Siderosis in the Bantu. A comparison of incidence in males and females. Bothwell TH, Isaacson C: The table

Am J Pathol 29:779–815 (1953) Siderosis in the Bantu of Southern Africa. Higginson J, Gerritsen MBTh, Walker ARP

J Lab Clin Med 58:845–853 (1961) Siderosis in the Bantu. The relationship between iron overload and cirrhosis. Isaacson C, Seftel HC, Keeley KG, Bothwell TH

Am J Clin Nutr 32:1272–1278 (1980) Changing patterns of dietary iron overload in Black South Africans. MacPhail AP, Simon MO, Torrance JD, Charlton RW, Bothwell TH, Isaacson C: Figures 1, 2, 3, and 4

S Afr Med J 53:365–368 (1978) The changing pattern of liver disease in South African Blacks. Isaacson C: Table 1 and 2

S Afr Cancer Bull 22:49–84 (1978) Cancer in the urban Blacks of South Africa. Isaacson C, Selzer G, Kaye Y, Greenberg M, Woodruff JD, Davies J, Ninin D, Vetten D, Andrew M: Tables 6, 7, 8, 9, 16, 29, 40, 41, and 42. Extensive use was also made of the material in the other tables

S Afr Med J 52:845–848 (1977) Idiopathic neurotrophic feet in Blacks. A pathological study. Isaacson C

S Afr Med J 55:413–415 (1979) Perinatal mortality in a Black urban community. Stein H, Mouton SCE: Table 1

References of Addendum to Chapters 5 and 6

Isaacson C, Paterson AC, Berson SD (1979) Hepatitis B surface antigen and hepatocellular carcinoma in Southern Africa. Virchows Arch (Pathol Anat) 285: 61–66

Kew MC (1981) Clinical, pathologic, and etiologic heterogeneity in hepatocellular carcinoma: Evidence from Southern Africa. Editorial: Hepatology 1:366–369

Kew MC, Desmyter J, Bradburne AF, Macnab BN (1979) Hepatitis B virus infection in Southern African Blacks with hepatocellular cancer. J Natl Cancer Inst 62:517–520

Kew MC, Ray MB, Desmet VJ, Desmyter J (1980) Hepatitis B surface antigen in tumour tissue and non-tumorous liver in Black patients with hepatocellular carcinoma. Br J Cancer 41:399–406

Paterson AC, Isaacson C (1982) Hepatocellular carcinoma in an urbanised black community: a changing pattern. Virchows Arch (Pathol Anat) (in press)
Shafritz DA, Kew MC (1981) Identification of integrated hepatitis B virus DNA sequences in human hepatocellular carcinomas. Hepatology 1:1–8
Shafritz DA, Shouval D, Sherman HI, Hadziyannis SJ, Kew MC (1981) Integration of hepatitis B virus DNA into the genome of liver cells in chronic liver biopsies and post-mortem tissue specimens. N Engl J Med 305:1067–1073

Subject Index

Index of Volumes 66–71 Current Topics in Pathology

Volume 66

Volume 67

Volume 68

Volume 69

Volume 70

Volume 71

MIX
Papier aus verantwortungsvollen Quellen
Paper from responsible sources
FSC® C105338
FSC
www.fsc.org

If you have any concerns about our products,
you can contact us on
ProductSafety@springernature.com

In case Publisher is established outside the EU,
the EU authorized representative is:
Springer Nature Customer Service Center GmbH
Europaplatz 3, 69115 Heidelberg, Germany

Printed by Libri Plureos GmbH
in Hamburg, Germany